LET'S TALK AB
MENTAL HEALTH AND
SAFETY

A manifesto for reducing mental injuries and suicides in, and caused by, the workplace

"Everyone (staff or contractor) deserves to go home from work mentally undamaged"

Copyright © 2020 by Nigel Bowker

FIRST EDITION

Dedicated to all those who have been the victims of mental injury at work and in particular those who have felt they have no alternative but to take their own lives.

May their future numbers be reduced.

CONTENTS

CHAPTER ONE

INTRODUCTION

This tome should never have been necessary. But in 2017 an event occurred which, apart from causing me real and lasting mental damage, has given me a valuable insight into how the world of work can be improved and even reduce the number of suicides. So once again I am writing a book.

A rule of presentations is to "tell them what you're going to tell them" so I'm going to follow that advice. Those of you with a short attention span might stop after that, but I'd like you to stay the course.

I start by telling my own story. Then I look at how the brain works and demonstrate that it can be damaged just as much as the rest of the body can be. I then look at the data for mental injuries and find there is no visible improvement. Neither is the frequency of suicides reducing.

I observe there is a lot of focus on mental health but, although necessary and worthy, it simply isn't sufficient. I then look for a model of success and discuss safety, where there has been a dramatic fall in UK work fatalities since the introduction of the Health and Safety at Work, etc. Act in 1974.

I then propose that we should adopt the concept of mental safety in the workplace and I demonstrate how the adoption of methods that have led to improvements in personal and process safety could similarly lead to improvements in mental safety. I demonstrate how this can be accomplished. I also take the opportunity to explain some of the principles of safety.

I don't claim to have found a magic bullet but I believe I have identified a way to considerably improve the situation in the workplace – and perhaps wider.

I don't know how many lives can be improved or saved by applying these principles but if it saves just one person from what I have suffered, my work will be worthwhile.

I have published this book as much as anything to promote discussion. I will be grateful for feedback on nigel@blackhallconsulting.co.uk.

I am more grateful than I can say to those who have taken the time to review the text: Audrey Bowker, Jen Bowker, Dianne Lamont, Alan Lamont, Jiwon Kim, Andrew Bowker, David Jamieson, Mark Bowker and Claire Rountree.

I would also be pleased to receive other examples and case studies, preferably with documentation.

Finally, if anyone has found this useful in their organisation or even implemented it, I would love to hear how it's gone!

CHAPTER TWO

THE BEGINNING OF A PERSONAL JOURNEY

This book isn't all about me. But had some events in 2017 not occurred, the book certainly wouldn't have been written. Furthermore, because those events have been so well documented by the companies involved, it also serves as a remarkable and indisputable case study as well.

So it seems reasonable to start by briefly recounting what happened.

By way of background, I am a chemical engineer with a work history that includes designing chemical and process plants; process plant operations; health, safety and environmental positions; and internal audit. Over a period of 32 years, I was employed by two firms of engineering design contractors and two of the world's largest oil companies. I retired from employment in 2008 and since then have been an independent consultant, specialising in applying and teaching process safety.

I am a Fellow of the Institution of Chemical Engineers (IChemE) and for three years I chaired the IChemE Aberdeen Member Group.

In my period as a consultant I worked extensively in collaboration with Company A. They had Company B as a client.

On 22nd February 2017 I was facilitating a HAZOP (a hazard and operability study)[1] for Company B via Company A. The meeting went perfectly fine from my standpoint, apart from a strange interjection from a person in Company B when I quoted a relevant comment my wife had made. He said "let's bin the misogyny". Misogyny was so far from the context of the situation, that I let his comment pass. That was my mistake. I would have been wise to have confronted him in the meeting because on 9th March 2017, my phone rang.

"Hello, Nigel, it's Mike. I don't know if you're aware, but there's been a complaint made against you."

---

[1] HAZOP is a method of systematically identifying hazardous events and significant operability issues emanating from within a process or utility system and ensuring they are appropriately mitigated.

Mike (who is not a villain in this story) was a contact at Company A.

My mind began to race. What on earth could this be? Had I accidentally submitted an incorrect invoice? What else could have led to a complaint? I had absolutely no idea what would come next.

"You've been accused of using misogynistic language," said Mike. He then read out the contents of an email, that I wasn't (and still am not) allowed to see, from Company B.

At that point, my world fell apart. I reviewed in detail what had happened at the meeting and knew that I had done nothing to cause offence. It was the beginning of great and continuing mental damage which my family, friends and I have had to live with ever since.

There was a lot of toing and froing thereafter. However, it's best that I tell the story in the indisputable words of the companies themselves, as communicated in letters in my possession. I have chosen to maintain the anonymity of the companies just now. But for context, Company A is a major engineering consultancy and Company B is an international oil company.

Under GDPR[2], I later obtained a letter from Company B to Company A dated 15th May 2017, stating:

"During the HAZOP, Mr Bowker made comments that were not in line with Company B values and behaviours and caused offence to other participants. On three occasions, Mr Bowker was asked by one of the participants to address his language but failed to do so." (Engineering Director, Company B)

This was clearly a serious allegation, which must have been carefully investigated.

I asked for the investigation report and received the following response:

"As Company B was not your employer, Company B did not conduct an investigation into allegations against you and therefore we do not

---

[2] General Data Protection Regulation. Its aim is to give people control over their personal data.

have any investigation report to send to you." (Director Workforce Concerns, Reporting & BI Transformation).

My goodness, I had been condemned in writing without any form of due process!

"Well", I hear you say, "Company A must have stood up for what was right?"

You'd imagine so, but on 26th May 2017 they wrote the following:

"Company B has undertaken a review of the incident ...... at Engineering Director level. Following Company B's discussions with the attendees, their finding is that you made comments that were not in line with Company B values and behaviours and caused offence to the participants. Company B advised Company A that on three occasions you were asked to address your language, but you failed to do so......... Company A supports Company B's findings in this matter." (Associate Director, Company A)

So what due diligence had they done to support Company B's findings?

".... We acted [on the information received] at face value." (Executive Vice President, Company A)

Is it acceptable for an engineering consultancy or indeed any professional company to take information from the client at face value?

Meanwhile, I have statements from or on behalf of all the meeting participants except the person who I know made the allegation that they (a) were not interviewed by Company A or Company B; and (b) not offended by anything I said. Indeed, I was congratulated on my facilitation. It took me ten minutes to obtain this information. Ten minutes that neither Company A nor Company B was prepared to spend to establish the truth.

So there you have it. Condemned by Company B on the basis of an unsubstantiated allegation. The allegation supported by Company A who took the allegation at face value. They had no interest whatsoever in hearing my point of view or in defending me despite my loyalty to them, even channelling significant projects to them. Did either company live up to their own values? Neither of them has apologised for their shortcomings or, so far as I am aware, dealt with the underlying issues.

Even as I write (July 2020) the CEO of Company B – who at the time of the allegation was head of the responsible division – chooses to ignore the facts by writing:

"Nigel – I understand that this issue was looked into by the team – and in line with standard practice – was referred to your employing company, Company A who handled it directly in accordance with their protocols. I'm sorry you are not satisfied with the outcome, but we wish you the best."

I can't fully describe the impact this had on me, but to have two well-regarded companies I had previously respected failing to have no regard for the truth – even in the face of evidence that they were wrong – pushed me deeply into depression.

What does it feel like? I am clinically depressed, I will be on medication for the foreseeable future and I am far from being the person I was before this event. It's a state of being physically alive but mentally numbed. Day and night there's a dark cloud in my brain. Suicidal thoughts have come into this clouded mind on more than one occasion.

However, as a long-term safety professional, I know that it's important to understand why things have occurred and how the world can be made better.

That is what I am seeking to do.

CHAPTER THREE

PERSUING THE THREAD

1. The brain

Clearly whatever changed to make me feel like this did so in my brain, so that has to be my starting point.

The brain is a remarkable organ, capable of almost unimaginable things. It consists of more than 100 billion nerves communicating through trillions of connections called synapses.

It contains many specialised areas that work together. On the outside is the cortex, which is Latin for "bark". It is frequently characterised as being made up of three types of zones: sensory, motor, and association areas. Thinking and voluntary movements begin in the cortex.

The brain stem links the brain to the spinal cord. It controls some basic functions such as breathing and sleep.

In the centre of the brain are the basal ganglia, which provide motor control, motor learning, executive functions and behaviours and emotions.

The cerebellum (Latin for "little brain") is near the brain stem and is responsible for coordination and balance.

The brain is also divided into several lobes. The frontal lobes are responsible for problem solving, judgment and motor function. The parietal lobes manage sensation, handwriting, and body position. The temporal lobes are involved with memory and hearing. The occipital lobes contain the brain's visual processing system.

So what happened to this beautiful piece of equipment to have led to my current state? I believe this is an area which isn't fully understood but it appears the mechanism is roughly as follows. The hippocampus is located near the centre of the brain. It stores memories and regulates the production of a hormone called cortisol. The body releases cortisol during times of physical and mental stress. If excessive amounts of cortisol are sent to the brain due to a stressful event or a chemical imbalance in the body this can lead to problems. In a healthy brain, neurons are produced throughout the adult life in a part of the hippocampus called the dentate gyrus. Long term exposure to increased cortisol levels can slow the production of new neurons and cause the neurons in the hippocampus to shrink. This puts you at increased risk of many health problems, including anxiety, depression, digestive problems, headaches, heart disease, sleep problems, weight gain and memory and concentration impairment.

PTSD (Post traumatic stress disorder) is caused through a similar process.

Some people are under the impression that their bad behaviour doesn't cause any actual damage to others and is therefore OK. They are wrong. It damages the brain. Everyone should be made aware of that. I call such events mental injuries.

You might say "But even if I recognise that brain damage is possible, not everyone will be damaged and those who are damaged won't be hurt in the same way." That is true but the same goes for other injuries. What we do in safety is to base our evaluations on what is credible.

But surely this is no problem, you can always have counselling or take anti-depressants and everything will be OK? In essence it's no worse than having to stick a plaster on a cut finger. Many anti-depressants such as Prozac (also known as Fluoxetine) are selective serotonin reuptake inhibitors (SSRIs). SSRIs affect your brain chemistry by slowing re-absorption of the neurotransmitter serotonin, a chemical that is thought to help to regulate mood and anxiety. Sometimes it works and sometimes it doesn't. I have been on Fluoxetine for quite a while now and believe me it hasn't restored me to my old self.

In any case, would it be satisfactory to cause people physical damage of any type on the basis that they can be repaired?

2.   The impact

What could the result of brain damage such as this be? There is no straight answer to this, any more than there would be if you ask me "what damage would I do to my car if I crashed it?". There is a range of possible outcomes, including:

- Nothing.

- Short term mental damage.
- Long term mental damage.
- Lost time associated with short or long term mental damage.
- Suicide.

To help us see how well as nation we are doing, we have detailed UK data for work-related stress, depression or anxiety, defined as a harmful reaction people have to undue pressures and demands placed on them at work. The latest data (rate per 100,000 workers) is shown below[3]:

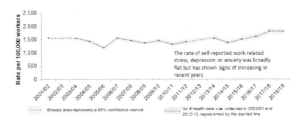

As the text on the chart says: "The rate of self-reported work-related stress, depression or anxiety was broadly flat but has shown signs of increasing in recent years."

This is a chart of estimated days lost (in millions):

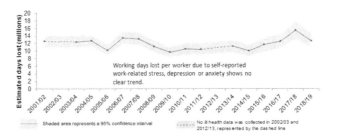

This is flat over the last 20 years, at best. These figures will be significantly worse than shown since many events are simply not reported. My own case wasn't reported, for example.

---

[3] Work-related stress, anxiety or depression statistics in Great Britain, 2019, Health & Safety Executive. Note that the link takes the reader to a document which is updated annually. It has been updated since I extracted the data from it. However, the new data just serves to reinforce my point.

The data is shown here by industry group:

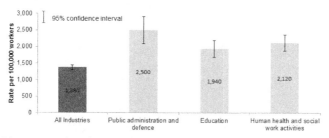

And by occupational category:

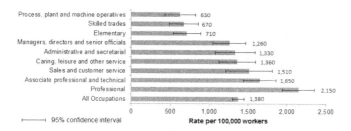

The professional occupations category has a statistically significantly higher rate than the rate for all occupations. For the three-year period averaged over 2016/17 to 2018/19 the professional occupations category had 2,150 cases per 100,000 people employed, compared with 1,380 cases for all occupational groups.

When we look at gender, women had statistically significantly higher rates compared with the average for all persons. This is evident in the ages ranges 25-54 years.

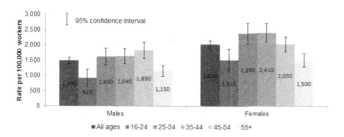

Let's talk about mental health and safety

Compared with the rate across all workplace sizes, small workplaces had a statistically significantly lower rate of work-related stress, depression or anxiety whilst large workplaces had statistically significantly higher rates. Medium sized work places weren't significantly different from the rate across all workplaces:

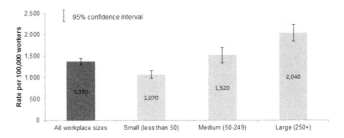

The data shown by cause or aggravation is:

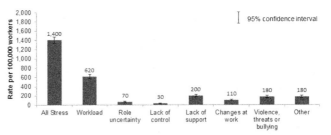

The Health & Safety Executive (H&SE) commentary is as follows:

- The total number of cases of work-related stress, depression or anxiety in 2018/19 was 602,000, a prevalence rate of 1,800 per 100,000 workers. This was not statistically significantly different from the previous period.

- The rate of work-related stress depression and anxiety was broadly flat but has shown signs of increasing in recent years.

- The number of new cases was 246,000, an incidence rate of 740 per 100,000 workers. The total number of working days lost due to this condition in 2018/19 was 12.8 million. This equated to an average of 21.2 days lost per case. Working days lost per worker due to self-reported work-related stress, depression or anxiety shows no clear trend.

- In 2018/19 these events accounted for 44% of all work-related ill health cases and 54% of all working days lost due to ill health.

- Stress, depression or anxiety is more prevalent in public service industries, such as education; health and social care; and public administration and defence.

- The main work factors cited by respondents as causing work-related stress, depression or anxiety were workload pressures, including tight deadlines and too much responsibility and a lack of managerial support.

So if we can address the frequency of mental injury we will improve lives and reduce lost time. This will benefit people and the economy. Estimates for the costs of mental issues vary widely but by way of example, the Centre for Mental Health suggests that mental health problems at work cost the UK economy £34.9bn (1.65% of GDP) in 2017.[4] It excludes the wider costs, such as the cost to the NHS. So, aside from other considerations, the size of the economic prize is clearly enormous.

3. Suicide statistics

In the extreme, these events can lead to suicide.

Unlike the data in section 2 above, there is no data for UK work-related suicides. However, let's work with what we have and see what we can learn.

Suicide statistics for the UK in 2018[5] were:

- There was a total of 6,507 suicides.
- Of these, 4,903 were men. This is 75% of the total and equivalent to 17.2 per 100,000 of the relevant population.
- 1,604 were women. This is 25% of the total and equivalent to 5.4 per 100,000.

---

[4] Mental health at work: The business costs ten years on, Michael Parsonage and Geena Saini, 5th September 2017.
[5] Suicide statistics report. Latest statistics for the UK and Republic of Ireland. December 2019. The Samaritans.

In 2019 things got even worse. The suicide rate for men in England and Wales was the highest for two decades.[6] Data from the Office for National Statistics (ONS) found there were 5,691 suicides registered in England and Wales, with an age-standardised rate of 11 deaths per 100,000 population.

Men accounted for about three-quarters of suicide deaths registered in 2019: 4,303 men compared with 1,388 women.

Rates have not fallen in the period from 2004. If anything, they have got worse. The Samaritans conclude:

> *"It is worrying to see a significant increase in suicide in the UK, for both men and women. Although, the overall increase seems to be driven by the rise in male suicide.*
>
> *Men remain around three times more likely to take their own lives than women in the UK. Middle aged men are still at greatest risk of suicide overall."*

People living in the most disadvantaged communities face the highest risk of dying by suicide. The Samaritans found that income and unmanageable debt, unemployment, poor housing conditions, and other socioeconomic factors all contribute to high suicide rates. They concluded that tackling inequality should be central to suicide prevention and support should be targeted at the poorest groups who are likely to need it most.[7]

The causes of suicide are many and complex, but it is clear that some of them are work-related and "some" is too many. It is disappointing that there is no record of how many UK suicides are caused or partially caused by work. Inquests may decide that a suicide is related to work but the data isn't correlated. There isn't even a record of how many suicides occurred in the workplace. In the USA the Bureau of Labor Statistics do record workplace suicides. These have shown an increase and a record number occurred in 2018. Workplace suicides don't equate to "work related suicides", of course. Neither are non-workplace suicides all non-work related.

---

[6] Suicides in England and Wales: 2019 registrations, Office for National Statistics.
[7] Socioeconomic Disadvantage and Suicidal Behaviour, Samaritans, March 2017.

20% of suicides in France are deemed to be work-related.[8]

A total of 1,748 people were killed in reported road traffic accidents in Great Britain in 2019.[9] Far more people die by suicide than are killed on the roads and yet road safety gets far greater funding than suicide prevention.

As mentioned earlier the impact on the UK economy is tens of billions of pounds. If we could reduce work-related lost time by 20%, that would benefit the economy by billions of pounds.

Let's further imagine that just 10%[10] of UK suicides had a work-related element. That would equate to 650 fatalities. Let's further imagine that we could cut that figure by 10%, i.e. 65 fatalities. Those are two prizes worth going after.

4.   Why are men so prone to suicide?

Male suicide rates are higher than women's around the world.[11] Some typical data is:

Country	Male suicide rate	Female suicide Rate
Argentina	15.1	3.5
Australia	19.5	7
Canada	18.1	7
France	23.9	11.7
Germany	19.7	7.7
India	17.8	14.7
Ireland	18.5	4.6
Japan	26	11.4
New Zealand	17.9	6.6
Russia	55.9	9.4
South Africa	18.7	4.7

---

[8] Suicidal work: Work-related suicides are uncounted, Sarah Waters, Hazards online special report, March 2017.
[9] Reported road casualties in Great Britain: provisional results 2019, Department for Transport, 30th July 2020.
[10] That would be half of the French assumption.
[11] https://worldpopulationreview.com/country-rankings/suicide-rate-by-country

Country	Male suicide rate	Female suicide Rate
South Korea	38.4	15.4
Spain	13.1	4.5
Sweden	19.1	10.5
United Kingdom	13.5	4.4
United States	23.6	7.2

Disappointing as things are in the UK, since we rank 78th globally on suicide rate, they are much worse elsewhere. Universally, though, men are more prone to suicide than women and by a large margin.

So to repeat the question, why are men more prone to suicide than women?

This is not quite as simple as it seems, as indicated by Helene Schumacher[12]. Her brother tragically committed suicide aged 28. Her research showed that in 2016 the World Health Organization (WHO) estimated there were 793,000 suicide deaths worldwide[13]. Approximately 63% were men.

She found the trend goes back a long way. "As long as we've been recording it, we've seen this disparity," says psychologist Jill Harkavy-Friedman, vice-president of research for the American Foundation for Suicide Prevention.

Schumacher found that women tend to have higher rates of depression diagnoses than men and are more likely than men to attempt suicide, but male suicide methods are often more violent, making them more likely to be completed before anyone can intervene.

Schumacher then hypothesised why men might be struggling. She concludes it's too simplistic to say women are willing to share their problems and men tend to bottle them up. But it is true that, for generations, many societies have encouraged men to be "strong" and not admit they're struggling.

---

[12] Why more men than women die by suicide, BBC Leader, 18th March 2019
[13] To put this in perspective, at the time of writing (October 2020) about a million people have died of COVID-19. In round number terms, that many people commit suicide every year.

The simple answer to the question might therefore be that men are more purposeful and successful at committing suicide, rather than more prone to the underlying conditions. This analysis is compatible with the injury data in section 2.

5. Can you be held responsible if an employee dies by suicide?

When a suicide occurs, it will automatically become the subject of an Inquest which will be required to look into the circumstances that culminated in the deceased's decision to take their life. Incidentally, inquests are very brief. Nick Spencer hanged himself at home on 7th April 2020 after been made redundant by bp. The inquest was programmed to take place from 10 am to 10.40 am on 30th September 2020[14]. It's difficult to see how deeply the coroner could have assessed the causes of this tragic event.

However, the inquest may decide that the suicide was work-related. This may in turn lead to criminal charges. It has always been possible to hold individuals possible for failures under health and safety legislation, but there was a growing desire to hold organisations and its senior management responsible. Hence, in 2007 the Corporate Manslaughter and Corporate Homicide Act was passed which could permit corporate prosecutions for work-related suicide, but to date there haven't been any such prosecutions under its banner.

Sarah Waters[15] tells us how it works elsewhere: "in France …. Workplace suicide is recognised officially in legislation and documented in government statistics. For instance, if a French employee takes his or her own life in the workplace, it is immediately investigated as a work-related suicide and the burden of proof is on the employer to demonstrate that the suicide was not work-related. Even if a suicide takes place outside of work, it is still considered as work-related if there is a connection with work – a suicide letter, a work uniform or use of a work implement. This presumption of causality is designed to protect the employee in an attempted suicide, or his or her family and circumvent the need for them to engage in legal action in order to prove the employer is liable."

---

[14] https://www.buckscc.gov.uk/services/births-deaths-marriages-and-civil-partnerships/coroner/buckinghamshire-forthcoming-inquests/
[15] Suicidal work: Work-related suicides are uncounted, Sarah Waters, Hazards online special report, March 2017.

There could also be a civil claim for negligence. A case that ran through the full English legal system is *Corr (administratrix of the estate of Thomas Corr deceased) v IBC Vehicles Ltd.* Mr Corr was employed as a maintenance engineer at IBC Vehicles Limited, a manufacturer of light commercial vehicles. On 22 June 1996 he was working on a prototype line of presses which produced panels for Vauxhall vehicles. He and a colleague were working to remedy a fault on an automated arm with a sucker for lifting panels. The machine picked up a metal panel from the press without warning and shunted it in Mr Corr's direction. He would have been decapitated if he hadn't instinctively moved his head. He was hit on the right side of his head, losing most of his right ear.

Mr Corr underwent long and painful reconstructive surgery. He remained disfigured, suffered persistently from unsteadiness, mild tinnitus and severe headaches, and had difficulty in sleeping. He also suffered from PTSD. He experienced severe flashbacks which caused his body to jolt and suffered from nightmares. He drank more alcohol than before the accident and became bad-tempered.

Mr Corr became depressed, felt life wasn't worth living and that he was a burden to his family. On 23 May 2002, while suffering from an episode of severe depression, he committed suicide by jumping from the top of a multi-storey car park.

His widow brought a claim for damages under section 1 of the Fatal Accidents Act 1976 (FAA). The FAA states "If death is caused by any wrongful act, neglect or default which is such as would (if death had not ensued) have entitled the person injured to maintain an action and recover damages in respect thereof, the person who would have been liable if death had not ensued shall be liable to an action for damages, notwithstanding the death of the person injured."

Mrs Corr argued her husband's physical and psychiatric injuries (including his suicide) were reasonably foreseeable consequences of the accident.

IBC Vehicles admitted that it had breached the duty of care it owed Mr Corr and that the breach caused the accident in 1996, but denied liability for his suicide.

The High Court dismissed Mrs Corr's claim. It held that although her husband's depression had been a foreseeable outcome of the accident, his suicide hadn't. They asserted that the question of reasonable foreseeability has to be judged at the time of the original accident, not with the benefit of hindsight. As Mr Corr hadn't had mental health problems before the accident, the company couldn't have foreseen that he would subsequently commit suicide.

The Court of Appeal, however, said that the question was not whether his suicide had been foreseeable but whether the kind of harm for which Mrs Corr was claiming damages (her husband's depression) was foreseeable. As the evidence clearly showed that the accident caused the PTSD which led to his depression and ultimately his suicide, there was no break in the "chain of causation" and Mrs Corr's claim could therefore succeed.

The House of Lords agreed. It said that personal injury included psychological injury and that Mr Corr's depression had been caused by his accident.

As a result of the accident "he acted in a way which he would not have done but for the injury." His suicide was therefore a foreseeable outcome of his injuries and the damages claimed fell within the scope of the duty that IBC owed Mr Corr.

They accepted that although "some manifestations of severe depression could properly be held to be so unusual and unpredictable as to be outside the bounds of what is reasonably foreseeable", suicide was not one of them.

As for the argument that his suicide had broken the "chain of causation", they said that "Mr Corr's suicide was not a voluntary, informed decision taken by him as an adult of sound mind making and giving effect to a personal decision about his future. It was the response of a man suffering from a severely depressive illness which impaired his capacity to make reasoned and informed judgments about his future ... It is in no way unfair to hold the employer responsible for this dire consequence of its breach of duty."

Nor was it necessary to make a finding of insanity before allowing a damages claim in such cases because suicide was no longer unlawful. The court declined to make a reduction for contributory negligence, saying it shouldn't attribute any blame to Mr Corr "for the consequences of a situation which was of the employer's making, not his". They were divided, though, as to whether reductions should be made in other such cases.

Note that although this was a physical injury, the court ruled that the psychological injury could reasonably have been foreseen.

So, be warned. Although ethics should guide you towards the sanctity of life and a concern to avoid harm, you can be held legally responsible for suicide.

CHAPTER FOUR

WHAT'S BEING DONE AND WHAT'S MISSING?

1. Mental health

Given that things aren't improving in the UK and many other countries as judged by either suicides or stress, depression and anxiety, what is the way of addressing it? "Mental health" is the normal answer and indeed organisations are keen to proclaim their support for mental health and have implemented programmes. The contents of these programmes, of course, differ widely. The UK H&SE has developed a set of Management Standards[16] which address:

- **Demands** – issues such as workload, work patterns and the work environment.

- **Control** – how much say the person has in the way they do their work.

- **Support** – this includes the encouragement, sponsorship and resources provided by the organisation, line management and colleagues.

- **Relationships** – this includes promoting positive working to avoid conflict and dealing with unacceptable behaviour.

- **Role** – whether people understand their role within the organisation and whether the organisation ensures that they do not have conflicting roles.

- **Change** – how organisational change (large or small) is managed and communicated in the organisation.

These correlate with many of the causes identified in Section 2 of Chapter 3.

---

[16] Tackling work-related stress using the Management Standards approach, H&SE, March 2019.

It will take time for the fruits of what is being done to show through, of course, but I intend to offer here a complementary approach.

This is especially pertinent for me given that Companies A and B both boast of their commitment to mental health and yet failed to show any concern for mine. This may well have been because I was a contractor but it's important that whatever you do extends across the workforce and isn't just limited to staff members. Everyone has the right to return home mentally undamaged by your business or activity.

I am not dismissing the wonderful efforts being made by many organisations in the current application of mental health, but I feel there is something missing. As I pondered this, I came across a historical analogy.

2. Is there a model world?

As a safety practitioner, my mind naturally turns to the world of safety and the tremendous progress that has been made.

This is a chart of fatal injuries to workers in Great Britain[17]:

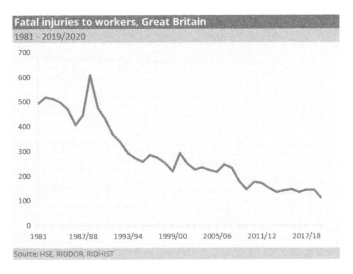

Fatal injuries to workers, Great Britain
1981 - 2019/2020

Source: HSE, RIDDOR, RIDHIST

---

[17] Health and Safety Statistics, Briefing Paper Number 7458, 21 July 2020, UK House of Commons.

Note this is absolute numbers of fatalities and the frequency will be falling even faster, given the growth in the workforce.

The following commentary was provided in the report:

> "This reduction is in part due to changes in the industry composition over the period (for example a shift away from mining, manufacturing and other heavy industry to lower risk service industries). A comparison of fatal injury numbers between 1974 (when the Health and Safety at Work Act was introduced) and 2018/19, adjusting to allow for the difference in industry coverage of the reporting requirements between these years, suggests that fatal injury numbers to employees have fallen by around 84% over this period."

So, even without correction, this is a pretty spectacular achievement. The comparison between this and suicides and non-fatal mental events is stark.

A historical analogy comes to mind. I live in Scotland and so pass to and fro across the Forth Estuary on a regular basis. There are three bridges within sight of each across the Forth at Queensferry.

The Forth (rail) Bridge was built by the Victorians. It was thought at the time that 57 lives had been lost building it. Recent research suggests this was more like 73.[18] Although no one thought this was excellent performance at the time, the project wasn't stopped. In the 1960s, the Forth Road Bridge was built at the cost of seven lives. More recently a third bridge – the Queensferry Crossing - has been built with only a single fatality. This is indicative of how society's expectations and industry performance have risen over the years with respect to personal safety.

On the subject of bridges, I can't move on without mentioning the Golden Gate Bridge in San Fransisco, constructed between 1933 and 1937. At the time there was an assumption that there would be one fatality for each million dollars of cost. That would have led to 35 fatalities. Joseph Strauss, the designer, wasn't happy with that and introduced many novel safety features. It was the first US construction site to make wearing a hard hat compulsory as was the

---

[18] https://www.scotsman.com/news/hidden-death-toll-forth-bridge-revealed-2467775

use of safety lines. Furthermore he spent $130,000 (over $2 million in today's money) on a safety net. The net saved nineteen lives. These survivors were known as the "Halfway to Hell" club. Although there were eleven fatalities this was a major landmark in safety performance. Ironically, ten of the fatalities were in a single event when a five ton work platform broke apart from the bridge and fell through the safety net. It shows both what a commitment to improvement can look like and how there is always more to do.

And, of course, we are all aware of the dramatic focus there has been on process safety in more recent years, spurred by notable disasters such as Piper Alpha, Texas City and Buncefield.

Mental health, however, is still stuck, relatively speaking, in the Victorian age.

Talking of mental safety and applying not just the existing mental health practices but many safety techniques could be the catalyst that is required.

At this point in the book, I have decided to pause and summarise my thoughts so far:

- Workplace stress events and all suicides are showing no reduction over a period of 20 years.

- Although there is an increased focus on mental health, this is showing no detectable improvement.

- On the other hand, the number of fatalities due to safety events has fallen dramatically over a long period of time.

- I recognise that the data is not directly comparable. However, it is the best information available.

- Furthermore, it is supported by my own experience at the hands of Companies A and B.

- This experience has also shown me that contractors are likely to have insufficient protection.

- Stress events have the potential to cause real physical changes in the brain – what I call mental injuries.

- We should:
    - consider mental injuries of equal importance to physical injuries;
    - talk of mental safety; and
    - apply more "safety" techniques to the mental health arena.

With this in mind, I want to:

- Encourage organisations the world over to build the protection of mental safety into their health and safety systems.

- Share some of the key health and safety concepts and tools that can be applied to the avoidance of mental injury.

- Encourage legislators and regulators to take mental safety more seriously – in a sense, to recognise that it is the next big barrier to reducing harm to people in the workplace.

3.   What do we mean by safety?

Safety is frequently mentioned, often out of scorn ("health and safety won't let us do it") and sometimes with impossible targets ("Things should be absolutely safe"). It is hence often misunderstood.

We often think that safety is a modern thing. Indeed, I may have reinforced that view with my use of the Forth bridges analogy. When the Pharaoh Khufu was having his pyramid built at Giza circa 2,500 BC it was necessary to move 6.5 million tonnes of rock. We have no idea how many people were killed and we tend to assume there was nothing in the way of safety requirements, let alone health policies.

Of course, we have no way of knowing, and we may do the ancients an injustice. As someone with a deep interest in history, I appreciate that the ancients were much more sophisticated than we often give them credit for. One indication of this comes from the code of Hammurabi. Hammurabi was a king of ancient Babylon between 1792 BC and 1750 BC or thereabouts. He inherited a small state and during his reign brought the whole of Mesopotamia under his rule. Mesopotamia was the ancient region of modern day Iraq between the Tigris and Euphrates rivers. It hosted many civilisations and empires including Ur, Akkad, Babylon and Assyria. Hammurabi is perhaps best known for his law code. A partial copy exists on a stone stele in the Louvre in Paris. It covers a wide range of legal aspects but specifically some directed at building safety:

If a builder builds a house for someone, and does not construct it properly, and the house which he built falls in and kills its owner, then that builder shall be put to death.

If it kills the son of the owner, the son of that builder shall be put to death.

If it kills a slave of the owner, then he shall pay, slave for slave, to the owner of the house.

If it ruins goods, he shall make compensation for all that has been ruined, and inasmuch as he did not construct properly this house which he built and it fell, he shall re-erect the house from his own means.

If a builder builds a house for someone, even though he has not yet completed it; if then the walls seem toppling, the builder must make the walls solid from his own means.

You will have noticed that all these criteria apply to the quality of the product, not to the safety of the workforce but nonetheless they are remarkable.

Let's now leap forward by 3,400 years to identify the origin of modern significant safety legislation. In the UK, the first such legislation was the *Health and Morals of Apprentices Act 1802*, introduced by Sir Robert Peel. This was followed by a number of factories acts but the next major step was the introduction of the *Factories Act* in 1833 which introduced a Factories Inspectorate.

A further major landmark was the passing of the *Health and Safety at Work etc. Act* in 1974. This was a revolutionary step as it brought all of health and safety within the UK under one Act. Under its umbrella, regulations (known as Statutory Instruments) can be enacted. Many of the requirements that we are familiar with day-to-day in the UK come to us via SIs, e.g the Health and Safety (Display Screen Equipment) Regulations 1992, also known as SI 1992 No. 2792.

Health and safety is often scorned in the UK but, as we have seen, since the introduction of the *Health and Safety at Work etc. Act,* there has been an 84% reduction in the number of fatal injuries.[19] How has this been achieved? One particular theory is that there have been three stages in the improvement:

- o **Stage 1** was a focus on equipment and engineering.
- o **Stage 2** was a focus on training and procedures.
- o **Stage 3** (the current stage) is a focus on behaviours.

The H&SE issue guidance notes for much of the health and safety legislation. They also, in collaboration with industry groups, develop Approved Codes of Practice (ACOPs) in certain areas. For example, lifting operations come under the banner of the *Lifting Operations and Lifting Equipment Regulations 1998 (LOLER)* which is supported by the *Lifting Operations and Lifting Equipment Regulations 1998. Approved Code of Practice and guidance.*

Legislation generally tends to be reactive, i.e. introduced after a problem has been identified or after a major disaster. A case in point is offshore safety. The Piper Alpha disaster in 1988 in which 167 people died led to major changes. The responsibility for offshore safety was moved from the Department of Energy (who had the responsibility until then since the installations concerned lie outside the three mile limit) to the H&SE. At the same time, the Safety Case Regulations[20] were introduced together with other associated legislation. This introduced the concept of safety cases for offshore oil and gas installations, bringing the offshore industry into line with high hazard onshore sites which come under the banner of the COMAH (Control of Major Accident Hazards) Regulations.

So, to revert to the title of this section "What do we mean by safety?" Wikipedia, that well known guide to everything, defines it as follows: "Safety is the state of being "safe" (from French sauf), the condition of being protected from harm or other non-desirable outcomes."

Legislation is seeking to impose this state of protection. How does this apply to mental safety, the subject of this book?

---

[19] Historical picture statistics in Great Britain, 2019. Trends in work-related ill health and workplace injury. H&SE, 30th October 2019
[20] Formally, the "Offshore Installations (Offshore Safety Directive) (Safety Case etc) Regulations". The latest edition became law in 2015 (SI 2015/398).

I use mental safety as a term to indicate prevention of mental damage to people, in the same way that "safety" is traditionally about the prevention of physical damage.

Where is this to be found in legislation? In the UK and many other countries, organisations have a duty of care to employees, contractors and volunteers. This includes providing a safe place of work including protection from mental damage. The latter point is not widely appreciated and so it is scarcely ever treated as equal with physical safety.

But at this point we can start to bring mental safety under the same umbrella as other health and safety effects, using the cause-consequence model:

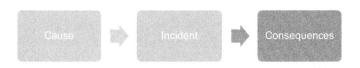

In this model, we recognise that a cause leads to an event, which in turn can have one or a range of consequences. Identifying this allows us to take appropriate action to eliminate or mitigate the event. We will return to this later.

However, meanwhile, let's develop a set of potential causes of mental damage. Here's a starter list:

- o Bullying.
- o Belittlement.
- o Limited participation in decision-making or low control over one's area of work;
- o Low levels of support for employees;
- o Inflexible working hours;
- o Unclear tasks or organisational objectives;
- o Overload;

  o Poor management and communication of organisational change.

Then it's important to understand the consequences. It helps to think in terms of damage. Most people understand what is meant by damage when we are dealing with "normal" safety. It leads to cuts, broken bones, even amputations and, most regrettably, even the occasional fatality or fatalities. These are the results we are trying to avoid or reduce the possibility of.

When it comes to mental damage, the results are not visible to an observer (excluding those equipped with brain scanners), although their effects can be. We don't need to get too much into the details but be constantly aware that the brain can be damaged by the way people are interacted with. This is one of the most crucial aspects of mental safety. The mental damage leads to other effects and, in the worst cases, suicide.

4. Models for health and safety

Over time, the concept of safety has developed two key areas. The first is **personal safety** or **occupational safety.** This is what most people think of when they hear the word "safety". It is focussed very much on protecting individuals or small groups from hazardous events. It includes matters such as:

  o Work control and permits.
  o Slips, trips and falls.
  o Dropped or falling objects.
  o Electrocution.
  o Falls from heights.
  o Vehicle accidents.

Typically one to three people might be at risk in a particular incident, although a major vehicle accident, for example, could cause significantly more fatalities. The risks can be much the same irrespective of the industry or locality. You can be the victim of a dropped object whether you work on a building site or a nuclear power station.

The other key category of safety is **process** or **technical safety**. This is where the materials used or the engineering can lead to a hazardous event. It includes matters such as:

    ○   Release of hazardous substances leading to asphyxiation, poisoning or fire and explosion.
    ○   Catastrophic technical failure.

The risks are therefore very dependent on the application. If there is no toxic inventory, you can't be poisoned.

For an example of the difference between these two types of safety, consider the aviation industry. When designing and manufacturing a new plane, you have the possibility of causing a major accident due to the plane disintegrating or crashing. This requires technical safety expertise. On the other hand, when assembling it you have to ensure the workforce don't get injured. This requires personal or occupational safety expertise. And you must never assume that you have "got" either type of safety. Boeing was founded in 1916 and has grown to be one of the world's biggest aircraft manufacturers. The Boeing 737 was launched in 1965. Since then, many variants have been produced. The latest version of the 737 is the 737 MAX. However, the design of the variant was disastrously bungled.[21] The errors made led to two fatal crashes with the loss of 346 lives. That is a technical safety failure. Ironically when you go to the Boeing website for an update on the 737 MAX you see them boasting of their commitment to Safety, Quality and Integrity.

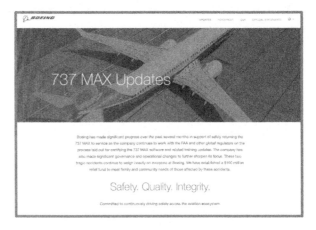

---

[21] Final Committee Report, The Design, Development and Certification of the Boeing 737 MAX, US Congress Committee on Transportation and Infrastructure September 2020.

To take the aircraft analogy further, design and manufacturing isn't enough. The manufacturer and the airline need to have a concern for the aircraft in service. The manufacturer needs to advise on any issues which it becomes aware of. The airline needs to have a focus on the ongoing technical integrity of the plane and the personal safety of the passengers, crew and maintenance personnel.

Hence, it has become commonplace to talk about lenses. We can look at safety through the lens of personal/ occupational safety or through the lens of process/ technical safety.

In some models, this is supplemented by a concern for mental health. So the model can be represented like this:

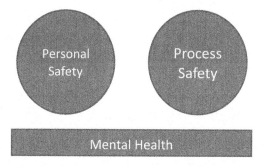

Mental health generally fails to deliver on the full mental safety agenda, as outlined previously. If evidence was required of this, just think of Companies A and B. They both claim to have a concern for safety and mental health and yet they were willing to ignore the reasonably foreseeable mental and financial injury that an unsubstantiated allegation would have on an individual. This isn't in any way to scorn mental health agendas, but I have amply demonstrated that what is being done is not enough and needs to be amplified and elevated in status. To put it another way, the mental health agendas are necessary but not sufficient.

I therefore propose promoting mental safety to the same level as personal safety and process safety to create a shamrock as follows:

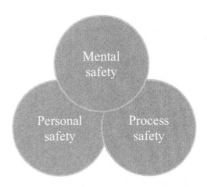

Indeed, it was originally intended to call this book "From Lens to Shamrock". This is far deeper, though, than just a modification to an illustration. It is about applying the same policies, procedures and methodologies to mental safety as to the rest of the safety agenda.

5.   Lack of consideration of mental safety

A lack of consideration for mental safety is rife. Unfortunately, many of these do not find their way into the public domain, especially when a financial settlement is reached covered by a non-disclosure agreement (NDA).

However, some well documented examples are worth noting:

Amnesty International. Two Amnesty International staff members died by suicide in 2018. A subsequent report[22] found that Amnesty International had a "toxic" working environment, with widespread bullying, public humiliation, discrimination and other abuses of power. It found a dangerous "us versus them" dynamic, and a severe lack of trust in senior management, which threatened Amnesty International's credibility as a human rights champion.

It added: *"As organisational rifts and evidence of nepotism and hypocrisy become public knowledge they will be used by government and other opponents of Amnesty's work to undercut or dismiss Amnesty's advocacy around the world, fundamentally jeopardising the organisation's mission."*

---

[22] Amnesty International Staff Wellbeing Review, Konterra Group, January 2019.

There have been a disappointingly large number of other suggestions of bad management behaviour (including bullying) across the UK charity sector.

France Telecom. Between January 2008 and April 2011 more than 60 France Télécom[23] employees died by suicide. 25 of these deaths occurred between 2008 and the early part of 2009. Some of the people left suicide notes blaming stress and misery at work. In December 2019 the former CEO Didier Lombard was found guilty of moral harassment towards his employees and sentenced to four months in jail.

NHS Highland and Argyll and Bute health and social care partnership. In September 2018, complaints were made about a culture of bullying at the NHS Highland Health Board in Scotland. A review was undertaken by John Sturrock QC who concluded it was possible that many hundreds of staff had been the victims of inappropriate behaviour. Many staff suffered serious harm and trauma as a result, driving them to quit their jobs or retire, although he stressed that it wasn't "possible to conclude conclusively that there is or is not a bullying culture in [NHS Highland]". [24]

As part of the response to this, NHS Highland undertook a survey in Argyll and Bute Health and Social Care Partnership (HSCP). 446 (29%) of the 1,540 NHS staff at Argyll and Bute HSCP responded to the independent survey, along with 62 former colleagues. 68% of the respondents indicated they had experienced bullying and harassment.[25]

All this is yet more evidence to my mind that we need to move on from talking just about mental health and start talking about mental safety.

---

[23] France Télécom is now Orange.
[24] Report to the Cabinet Secretary for Health and Sport into Cultural Issues related to allegations of Bullying and Harassment in NHS Highland, April 2019, John Sturrock QC.
[25] Argyll & Bute Health and Social Care Partnership Culture Review – Survey results – Summary. Commissioned by NHS Highland in partnership with Argyll & Bute Health and Social Care Partnership May 2020.

CHAPTER FIVE

IMPLEMENTING MENTAL SAFETY

1. The basics

Let's assume that you have been convinced by my line of reasoning and decided to formally implement mental safety.

Let me ask you two questions about your company or organisation:

Q1: Do you have a commitment to physical safety? – if so, what evidence can you provide?

Q2: Do you have a commitment to mental safety? – if so, what evidence can you provide?

Most people can provide enormous amounts to support the answer "yes" for the first question. When it comes to the second question, though, there is a struggle to find anything comparable in the way of evidence.

Why is this? Most organisations have never considered their responsibility for mental safety.

How can this be reversed? My original idea was to develop a set of commitments and I will outline a set of those soon, but I am now inclined to think that first of all you should become introspective and do these two things:

- **Conduct a staff survey using a questionnaire.** Some typical questions might be:
  - Does the organisation care about mental safety as much as physical safety? If not, what are the differences?
  - Have there been any incidents that have led to mental damage? If so, what were they?
  - Have you been trained in mental safety?
  - Do you consciously apply mental safety in your interactions with people?
  - Do you have mental safety targets?
  - Are you assessed in your delivery of mental safety?
  - Does your direct superior demonstrate concern for mental safety?

---

o Is there any difference in the way that staff and non-staff personnel are treated with respect to mental safety?

o Are mental injuries reported and investigated?

o Have you known the organisation engage in "trade offs" against mental safety?

o Do the victims of mental injury receive the same degree of medical care as the victims of physical injuries?

o Have you seen any retribution against those who report mental injuries?

o Does the organisation insist that its contractors respect mental safety?

o Does management take responsibility for mental safety?

  ▪ Do they collect and assess data to determine the current state of safety?

  ▪ Do they implement controls?

  ▪ Have they ever recognised a breach of those controls?

o Who is responsible for the mental safety policies and are they suitably independent from managers?

o Is there an internal review of the policies and a check on the efficacy of the controls?

The actual questionnaire might include scoring to enable prioritisation of actions and periodic review.

- **Examine your absence data and determine how much of it is associated with mental safety issues**. Ideally, you will have logged these already in your accident and incident reporting system and developed the lessons learned – but that may be wishful thinking.

2. Commitments

Now to developing some commitments. You should create your own list but here's a default one which can be supplemented by the results of the staff survey and lessons derived from the absence data.

1. We will treat mental safety as equal in importance with personal safety and process safety.

2. We will develop and enforce standards of conduct for protecting mental safety.

3. We will train our management and workforce in mental safety.

4. We will include mental safety targets in company and personal objectives.

5. We will assess employees in their delivery of mental safety.

6. We will not differentiate between staff members, contractors and visitors regarding mental safety. Everyone deserves to go home undamaged mentally.

7. We will have a system of reporting mental injuries.

8. We will investigate mental injuries with the same rigour as physical injuries.

9. We will never engage in arbitrary "trade offs" against mental safety.

10. We will ensure that the victims of mental injury receive the same degree of medical care as the victims of physical injuries.

11. There will be no retribution against those who report mental injuries.

12. We will impose similar requirements on our contractors.

I will now go on to discuss these commitments one by one.

Commitment 1: "We will treat mental safety as equal in importance with personal safety and process safety."

Why is it necessary to say this? Simply because the risk of mental injury isn't on the health and safety agenda for many organisations. To date, the financial cost to many organisations of causing mental injury is inconsequential compared with the cost of causing a physical injury to an individual. Relevant policies such as harassment, bullying and equality rest with the HR department, and are not subject to rigorous implementation controls. Regard for mental safety is not part of the management agenda as physical injuries and process safety are.

A positive approach would be to adopt the Shamrock Model and move to build mental safety into corporate processes. Clearly, your mental health system becomes a part of the mental health and safety system, but there will be gaps to be filled.

We spend a lot of time working out how people can be physically injured at work or how process safety events can occur – and put the appropriate number of controls in place - but pay less attention to how people can be subject to mental injury and ensuring they are adequately protected.

One of the important things about moving from a discussion of mental health alone to mental health and safety is the reality that we have the capacity to physically damage people's brains in the same way that we can damage people's bodies. This is a leap in perspective and management should seek to understand this, using in house medical expertise or seeking external assistance.

Commitment 2: "We will develop and enforce standards of conduct for protecting mental safety."

How often have we heard bad behaviour justified on the basis of passion, focus, "management have the right to manage" or other trite phrases?

Such terms are used almost continuously not only in business and voluntary organisations but even by government ministers and advisors as justification for how they behave.

Dominic Cummings is a key character in current British politics. To call him controversial would be something of an understatement. He led the 2016 "Vote Leave" campaign to take the UK out of the European Union. When Boris Johnson became prime minister in July 2019 Cummings was appointed his chief advisor. He was credited in large measure with masterminding Johnson's subsequent overwhelming election victory in December 2019. Cummings believed that Sonia Khan, a special adviser in the Treasury, had been dishonest about her recent contact with Philip Hammond, the previous Chancellor of the Exchequer. It appears that Cummings made allegations to her, sacked her without any due process and had her escorted out of 10 Downing Street by an armed police officer. In a subsequent meeting with the special advisers, Cummings is alleged to have to have said: "If you don't like how I run things, there's the door." Clearly, his 'right to manage' was paramount and apparently legitimised his actions. Perhaps it's too much for our political classes to model good behaviour. It's reported that Ms Khan received compensation of £50,000 to £100,000[26]. It's not known what mental damage she suffered.

Another example from UK politics is Pritti Patel, the current[27] UK Home Secretary. Patel is another robust character. Her husband Alex Sawyer apparently calls her "my personal piranha" because she's small and combative. Patel's permanent secretary resigned claiming constructive dismissal. This has now gone to an employment tribunal. It is the first time that a secretary of state has been pursued to an employment tribunal by a former permanent secretary, the most senior civil servant in a government department. His case is expected to focus on claims that in late 2019 and early 2020 he challenged Patel's alleged mistreatment of senior civil servants in the Home Office, and that he was then hounded out of his job through anonymous briefings. Patel was the subject of a seven-month Cabinet Office inquiry which concluded she had breached the Ministerial Code, even if she wasn't aware she was bullying staff. The prime minister then concluded Patel hadn't breached the code and shouldn't resign. This is a very British muddle and a backward step for mental safety. It simply isn't acceptable for politicians to throw their weight around on the basis of having a "mandate from the people" as if they are above the law. Such matters should be dealt with as safety issues, which is what they are.

It is true that management have the right to manage but they have the obligation to do it within acceptable boundaries and not to follow the mantra of "the end justifies the means"[28].

Quite simply, if we aren't aware of the need to avoid mental injuries, the possibility of them will play no part in many people's decision making and actions. We need to place boundaries around acceptable behaviour. Many of these boundaries are well-known, common sense and indeed simple morality. However, there are too many cases of them being ignored. Bullying, victimisation, discrimination and belittlement are all too common at all levels.

---

[26] The Times, 13th November 2020.
[27] As at October 2020.
[28] This expression may originate in Ovid's Heroides (1st century BC). The poem contains a line that can be translated as the result justifies the deed or the ends justify the means.

I reiterate – and make no apology for it - that it's important for people to have an awareness of the real physical harm that can be done to the brain through repeated or unresolved abuse of any kind.

Commitment must be genuine and heartfelt.

Sometimes organisations need pressure to do the right thing and so stakeholders have a role to play.

- **Shareholders** (especially the major investing institutions such as pension funds) should see this an important matter of social responsibility. Shareholder pressure has contributed in very large measure to companies taking climate change seriously and shown the power of the large investment institutions in particular. In 2020 Rio Tinto committed an act of archaeological and sociological vandalism by blasting aboriginal sacred sites at Juukan Gorge in Australia. Eventually shareholder unease led to the Chief Executive and other senior managers leaving the company.[29] Imagine what could happen if shareholders expressed a meaningful concern for mental safety.

- **Regulators**, too, should be involved. I struggle to find an example of the UK Health & Safety Executive recommending a prosecution for failure to protect mental safety. All it would take would be one high focus prosecution to get the attention of management and establish mental safety firmly on corporate agendas.

- **Governments and legislators** can also assist, either through legislation or by publicly holding managers to account for their shortcomings through parliamentary committees and questions in parliament. I need at this point to pay credit to Theresa May, the former UK prime minister, who created the new role of Minister for Suicide Prevention and Mental Health in the Department of Health and Social Care.

---

[29] "Rio Tinto Executive Committee changes", Rio Tinto press release, 11 September 2020.

A suicide prevention strategy has been established in England, focusing on seven key areas:[30]

- o Reducing the risk of suicide in high risk groups.
- o Tailoring approaches to improve mental health in specific groups.
- o Reducing access to means of suicide.
- o Providing better information and support to those bereaved or affected by suicide.
- o Supporting the media in delivering sensitive approaches to suicide and suicidal behaviour.
- o Supporting research, data collection and monitoring; and
- o Reducing rates of self-harm as a key indicator of suicide risk.

The Scottish government has also established a series of priorities:[31]

- o Setting up and funding a National Suicide Prevention Leadership Group (NSPLG).
- o Funding the creation and implementation of refreshed mental health and suicide prevention training.
- o Working with the NSPLG and partners to encourage a coordinated approach to public awareness campaigns, which maximises impact.
- o With the NSPLG, ensuring that timely and effective support for those affected by suicide is available across Scotland by working to develop a Scottish Crisis Care Agreement.
- o The NSPLG will use evidence on the effectiveness of differing models of crisis support to make recommendations to service providers and share best practice.
- o The NSPLG will work with partners to develop and support the delivery of innovations in digital technology that improve suicide prevention.
- o The NSPLG will identify and facilitate preventative actions targeted at risk groups.
- o The NSPLG will ensure that all of the actions of the Suicide Prevention Action Plan consider the needs of children and young people.
- o Work closely with partners to ensure that data, evidence and guidance is used to maximise impact. Improvement methodology will support localities to better understand and minimise unwarranted variation in practice and outcomes

---

[30] Preventing Suicide in England, Third progress report of the cross-government outcome strategy to save lives, January 2017.
[31] Scotland's Suicide Prevention Action Plan.

o   Work with the NSPLG and partners to develop appropriate reviews into all deaths by suicide, and ensure that the lessons from reviews are shared with NSPLG and partners and acted on.

It would be good to see these plans implementing the principles of mental safety, especially in organisations.

- **Unions** can contribute too. For example, this is a press release by the UK union Unite concerning the proposed appointment of a new CEO (Jeremy Hughes) by the Samaritans:

> "Unite, the UK and Ireland's largest union, is calling on the trustees of the Samaritans to reverse their decision to appoint Jeremy Hughes as the charity's new chief executive.
>
> The union which represents around 50 staff at the charity made its call after several stories emerged about the behaviour of Mr Hughes during his present tenure as chief executive of the Alzheimer's Society, resulting in £750,000 being spent on non-disclosure agreements (NDAs).
>
> Unite is especially concerned about Mr Hughes' management style as the union has had to represent a large number of members who were subjected to bullying at the Samaritans by former members of its management team."

Unite regional officer Peter Storey said:

> *"The revelations about Mr Hughes are deeply troubling. Given the fact that the Samaritans is in the very early stages of recovering from a toxic bullying culture which has damaged the lives of many of its staff, Unite does not believe that Mr Hughes is the right person to heal the problems the charity has experienced.*
>
> *Unite believes it is incumbent on the trustees at the Samaritans to rescind the appointment of Mr Hughes as its chief executive and instead appoint someone who has a track record in tackling a toxic bullying culture.*
>
> *Unite's members at the Samaritans are absolutely dedicated to the excellent work that the charity undertakes and they*

deserve to perform their roles in a healthy and respectful environment."

The appointment was cancelled. Incidentally, how appalling is it that the Samaritans could even be suspected of permitting bullying? I mean who do you call if you are considering suicide and you work for the Samaritans?

The UK Trades Union Congress has issued a paper called "Work and Suicide"[32] which seeks to mobilise various stakeholders.

- And, of course, **Consumers** can play their part by refusing to deal with organisations that have not implemented mental safety into their business processes.

All, in all, it's perhaps not too much to say, though, that there is a form of abuse that is all-too-often secretly condoned in our society.

Commitment 3: "We will train our management and workforce in mental safety."

But surely everyone is trained in safety? Yes, but that tends to be personal safety and sometimes process safety. Although many companies provide mental health training, it generally includes little or nothing on how people can be mentally injured at work. The example of NHS Highland - almost unbelievably - highlights how even a health authority can fail to recognise at senior levels how management behaviour can lead to mental damage.

Furthermore, we typically apply few of the other safety techniques to mental safety. For example, how often do we apply the principles of cause → consequence → safeguard, or do risk assessments, or apply barrier models, or conduct investigations when mental safety is damaged? Incidentally, if you're not familiar with all these expressions, read on!

People from the top down need to be aware of when actions or events can lead to mental injuries and ensure the cause is eliminated or the likelihood is tolerably low, as with other aspects of safety.

---

[32] TUC, Work and Suicide, 27 February 2019.

It is no wonder that mental injuries continue to occur at a worrying rate.

So implementing a programme of mental safety cannot just be done by issuing a memo or an email. It will involve enormous cultural change, often in the face of generations of accepted practice and making it plain to management that some of the characteristics that helped them into their current positions will have to change if they want to remain there.

It will involve the same long, hard but successful journey we took to improve safety. There is a famous photograph ("Lunch atop a skyscraper") showing eleven men eating lunch, sitting on a girder with their feet dangling 840 feet (260 metres) above the New York City streets. The photograph was taken on 20th September 1932 on the 69th floor of the RCA Building during the last months of construction. Although it looks ad hoc, the photograph was staged for publicity to promote the new skyscraper. Other photographs taken on the same day show some of the workers throwing a football and pretending to sleep on the girder. It's unlikely that anyone would think this a suitable publicity photograph if staged today. In those days most skyscraper projects had fatalities. Fatalities would be the exception today.

Similarly, if we are to replicate with mental safety the improvement in occupational safety, training is required and that training must begin at the top. This shows genuine commitment.

What form will this training take? Well, that depends. Mental safety shouldn't be treated differently from other safety matters, but it must be treated as equal. By this I don't mean just slipping in the words "mental safety" as a token gesture, of course. The training should emphasise the real and permanent damage that can be done to the brain by the way we relate to people and how that can lead to permanent disability and even death, just as a physical injury can.

Commitment 4: "We will include mental safety targets in company and personal objectives."

Given that mental issues are so high profile, how many companies have developed targets for mental safety in the same way that they have for personal safety and process safety? In truth, I have never come across a company or organisation that has a set of measures specifically related to mental safety.

There's a well-known business cliché "What gets measured gets done". (The quotation is often attributed to Peter Drucker but the authors of Geography Matters! suggest it may go back to the Renaissance astronomer Rhaticus who said that if you can measure something, then you have some control over it). Although this is somewhat simplistic – after all, we can all think of many things that get measured without being done – it is more likely true that what doesn't get measured is left to serendipity.

What form might these measures take? We generally think in terms of two types of performance measures:

- o   Input measures (sometimes called leading indicators).
- o   Output measures (sometimes called lagging indicators).

We sometimes add a third type called "process measures".

Input measures are those things we do to influence performance. Output measures look at results.

Clearly input measures are best since they prevent bad things from happening. Too many organisations only measure outputs.

So what might be some suitable inputs for mental safety? Here are some initial thoughts:

- o   The number of staff trained in mental safety.
- o   The number of people with mental safety targets in their job description or annual objectives.
- o   The number of appraisals conducted that discuss mental safety.
- o   The number of audits undertaken into mental safety application.

And what might be some suitable outputs?

- o   Fatalities (suicides) attributable to work-related mental injuries.
- o   The number of mental safety incidents logged.
- o   The number of workdays lost due to mental safety issues.
- o   The cost of mental safety workdays lost.
- o   Staff survey results.
- o   The number of enforcement actions taken by regulators for mental safety failures.

o   The number of prosecutions for mental safety failures.

My extensive experience in seeing other safety systems implemented has shown the importance of honesty. Management need to be prepared to log mental safety events and treat the reporting itself as being good. No attempt should be made to cover up reporting; indeed, it should be encouraged. Because of this, in the early stages of implementing a programme, performance may seem to be deteriorating, but this can often be good news in disguise, as people get more confident about reporting events. It allows a kind of baseline to be established, from which genuine improvement can be seen. Furthermore, it develops confidence in the workforce that the commitment is genuine.

Most organisations report on the health and safety performance whether it be within their annual report or in a separate sustainability report or both. In many cases, there are detailed statistics for personal and, where applicable, process safety and environmental performance. And then there are at best a few words about mental health.[33] This helps to show the relative ranking of these matters in the minds of the leadership.

Commitment 5: "We will assess employees in their delivery of mental safety."

Most organisations undertake staff appraisals. This should include mental safety. When should assessment start? Earlier than you might think and ideally at the recruitment stage. Someone with a track record of bad behaviour is unlikely to change no matter what fine words they might use at the interview. A behavioural track record can be difficult to determine but often some subtle enquiries can be made. This is particularly possible when recruiting at senior levels since it can form part of the executive search process. One wonders what enquiries the Samaritans made when recruiting their CEO as referred to previously. Given the nature of their work, one would hope they would be particularly sensitive to the possibility of a CEO causing mental damage. The use of non-disclosure agreements (NDAs) can also be a clue. Obviously by their nature NDAs are meant to be confidential but their existence (if not the details) can often be an open

---

[33] See, for example, the bp Sustainability Report 2019,
https://www.bp.com/content/dam/bp/business-
sites/en/global/corporate/pdfs/sustainability/group-reports/bp-sustainability-
report-2019.pdf

secret, as we have seen. Sometimes when making an appointment it is necessary to apply some conditions. A person may be a perfect fit in many ways for a job and yet have some behavioural gaps. If it's felt the individual would be capable of stepping up to the plate (and that can be tough to assess), an action plan (the use of coaching, for example) can form part of the appointment.

Having made wise recruitment choices, corporate and individual targets for mental safety should be developed. Then, it's important that performance against these targets is assessed during the appraisal system.

This is, of course, crucially dependent on appropriate training having been provided.

Appraisals should be honest and lead to the development of useful areas for improvement. This may include additional training or coaching.

Commitment 6: "We will not differentiate between staff members, contractors and visitors regarding mental safety. Everyone deserves to go home undamaged mentally."

This of course is very poignant to me since both Company A and Company B regarded me as having a different status because I was not a staff member with either of them. Indeed, if I had been employed by one or other of these companies, the matter would most likely have been properly addressed and my mental injury wouldn't have occurred.

When I worked as an Offshore Production Engineer in the Forties Field in the late 1980s, a production supervisor came into my office one day to advise me that someone had been sprayed with some chemicals from an oxygen scavenger[34] hose that had been left on the deck without being properly drained. He then felt it necessary to say "But don't worry, it's only a contractor." I looked him in the face and said "Don't forget that contractors are people too". In return, I got a look of complete incomprehension. That wasn't such an unusual ethos in those days.

---

[34] Oxygen scavenger was pumped into the injection water to remove residual oxygen to prevent corrosion and bacterial growth.

Things have improved in many ways regarding companies facing up to their health and safety obligations towards contractors since then but it is still imperfect. Companies generally do care more about contractors especially where they are working on a site where the company is the legal Duty Holder.[35] When I say that things have improved, I am not of course talking about mental safety since most organisations have an inadequate concept of it, whether it be to staff or contractors.

The legal duty of care doesn't just extend to people working on your site. If you cause an injury anywhere, you can be held responsible and this should be applied also to mental safety since it is different to personal or process safety.

Overwhelmingly you need to believe – and display – that everyone (staff, contractors and others) deserve to go home from work mentally undamaged.

Organisations must never confuse the employment status of a contractor with their health and safety rights.

Commitment 7: "We will have a system of reporting mental injuries."

Every personal injury from a fatality down to a "no treatment" event is logged and investigated in responsible organisations.

Yet, how many organisations even have a way of identifying each and every mental safety event, let alone logging and investigating them?

To report mental injuries you have to recognise them. This requires the organisation to have an open reporting system where someone who has been the victim of a mental safety incident feels able to report it without fear of retribution. Even more, other people need be trained to recognise that an event has taken place. Achieving this depends on having a deep-seated cultural change. This highlights the importance of a move towards caring about mental safety starting with cultural change led from the top.

---

[35] The Health and Safety at Work Act describes the Duty Holder as the person "who has, to any extent, control of premises". This may be a real person or a "virtual person" known as a persona ficta in legal terms, such as a corporate body.

Any retribution taken should, of course, be dealt with firmly and using the corporate disciplinary system.

When the company I then worked for was introducing a behavioural safety system in the early 1990s, a brave soul had to point out to the senior management that they were out of step with the new behaviours. To do the management justice, they issued a note admitting they'd had a "wake-up call" and brought in a management coach to help them. The move towards caring for mental safety requires the same openness and degree of humility.

Commitment 8: "We will investigate mental injuries with the same rigour as physical injuries."

In the case of any physical injury or near miss, we investigate it.

How do we do this? First of all we set up a team, the composition of which will depend on the nature and actual or potential severity[36] of the event. Team members should have had incident investigation training and at least one member should have specialist expertise, especially in root cause analysis. Each investigation should have a terms of reference. A serious incident such as a fatality should be led by a senior executive with no linkage to the event. Sometimes help is required from outside the organisation.

Many forms of commercial incident investigation systems are available, but it isn't necessary to use fancy software to get a decent result.

The team sets out to establish first the timeline of the event, including any relevant history.

As they probe backwards and forwards through time they will be able to identify the immediate causes of the event. Often people will stop at this point but it's important to enquire further. This allows us to identify the underlying or root causes.

Let's take an example from the area of safety. A report comes in that someone has been injured in a workshop and the injured party has

---

[36] The incident might have resulted in no injury but under other reasonably foreseeable circumstances it might have led to much more serious consequences. It needs to be investigated as if the more serious outcome had occurred so the lessons can be learned.

been taken to hospital. You establish an investigation team and issue them with a terms of reference. They visit the workshop where they take copies of all the relevant documentation, including procedures and permits, and take photographs.

The team then interview all the people in the workshop. Then they are advised the injured party is well enough to be interviewed in hospital so they do that.

What they discover is that an object was being lifted in the workshop using an overhead crane. Suddenly, the object fell to the ground, impacting the injured party on the way to the ground. The person wasn't involved in the lifting operation but was just making his way across the workshop floor. He sustained a broken leg but the injury could have been a lot more serious. He could credibly have been killed.

The team determine that there were two immediate causes of the accident:

1.   The object fell.
2.   The person was in the area.

They then seek to establish the historical timeline to understand how both of these matters came about. Post-it Notes (or equivalent) can be useful for constructing the timeline.

For the falling object, they discover that the clutch on the crane failed. They probe further back and determine that the previous clutch had been replaced six months before. The age of the crane meant that an exact replacement wasn't available but a similar one had been fitted. Unfortunately, there was an incompatibility between the crane and the clutch which lead to accelerated wear on the clutch plates and the subsequent failure.

So they concluded that the wrong component had been fitted. Job done! Well, no.

They had determined what had happened but not **why** it happened. So they carried on probing. They reviewed why this incompatible piece of equipment had been fitted. They discovered the maintenance supervisor had conducted a cursory review and concluded that it would fit, which was his main concern. It wasn't reviewed by a technical authority and crucially wasn't authorised via the organisation's management of change system since it was decided that it really wasn't a change, just a replacement.

So, the investigation went from a dropped object into the guts of the way the organisation managed change and found it to be poorly understood and applied. Why was this? Management regarded it as being just a piece of process and the staff hadn't been trained in its use. Now deeper realities were emerging about management commitment.

So, in conducting an investigation you probe back through each line of enquiry until there is nothing further to identify.

One approach to this is the *five whys* method. It was invented by Sakichi Toyoda who started the Toyoda group of companies, which includes Toyota, founded by his son. In applying the *five whys* you simply keep on asking "why?" until you get to the underlying root cause. Now, it has to be said there's nothing magical about the number five here. It just happens to be a number which frequently gives the right answer. Applied to our case, it could be as follows:

The problem: The wrong clutch was fitted.

1. Why? The supervisor thought it would be OK.
2. Why? It hadn't been properly evaluated.
3. Why? It hadn't been passed through the management of change system.
4. Why? People hadn't been trained in the use of the MOC system.
5. Why? Management weren't committed to the MOC system.

As you can see, this can be a very powerful tool.

The second immediate cause of the incident was that the injured party was in the potential drop area. This too was investigated by the team. They found that there was a walkway running under the drop area. Some time before it had been identified that when lifting operations were taking place, the walkway should be barriered off. This wouldn't cause significant inconvenience since there was another walkway.

As they investigated this, they found that the procedure hadn't been followed since its development. They further found that in general there was no awareness of procedures and hence they weren't applied. The root cause was once again management commitment.

Properly conducted investigations lead not just to the root cause of the issue in question but to deeper truths within an organisation. From there, a series of meaningful recommendations can be made that address far more than just the incident in question.

We need to apply it to mental safety if we are to make progress.

On 25 July 2013, Rhys Connor, 25, hanged himself in his room at the Hope Downs mine site in the Pilbara in Western Australia whilst working fly-in-fly-out (FIFO)[37] for Rio Tinto. Rio Tinto didn't investigate his death since it wasn't on the worksite. However, had they done so they would have learned a number of important lessons, including the fact that Rhys intentionally kept his depression secret from his employer OTOC. This was a lost opportunity to learn lessons and who knows there might have been a previous event that, had it been acted upon, would have prevented this one?

In our case study, neither Company A or Company B undertook even the most cursory of investigations. Had either of them bothered to do so little as to speak to the people I had supposedly caused distress to, they would have discovered this was a fabricated allegation, which through ignorance they both went on to support. This would have taken them perhaps ten minutes. Furthermore, they would have discovered that the person who made the allegation had a history of making allegations.

What's even more concerning is that neither company benefited from the deeper lessons from this, such as the importance of adopting the principles of mental safety.

But no matter. It wasn't a safety matter so far as they were concerned.

This demonstrates another important reason for undertaking investigations in the pursuit of mental safety: the search for truth. The truth is important when undertaking all investigations, of course, since unless we are clear about the facts we can't get to the root causes

---

[37] Fly-in fly-out (FIFO) is a method of flying people into remote work areas temporarily instead of relocating them and their families permanently. It's common in large mining regions in Australia and Canada.

and make meaningful recommendations. In the case of mental safety, getting clarity about the facts can also be important in <u>preventing</u> events occurring in the first place, such as by the making of false allegations.

Commitment 9: "We will never engage in arbitrary "trade offs" against mental safety."

When there is the risk of a physical injury or a physical injury has actually taken place, there is no debate as to what happens. In the former case, a risk assessment will be undertaken to ensure that the precautions taken are compatible with the potential consequences. In the latter case, appropriate responses are taken to prevent recurrence. Whether the person is an employee or a contractor, ethical and law abiding organisations will stand up for what is right in terms of providing medical assistance and investigating the event.

This is generally not the same with mental injuries. Organisations feel free to play a game of denial and pursuit of their own short term commercial or other objectives. It can be made plain – as in our case study – that these are best served by not embarrassing their client. "Don't rock the boat" can be the mantra. Indeed three years after the event Company A was awarded a new global framework agreement (contract) by Company B, so what they did was amply rewarded in their eyes.

This has echoes of some of the worst days of personal safety not so many years ago when contractors would routinely be leaned upon to keep injury statistics down.

It is only by standing up for what is right that a commitment to mental safety can gain credibility and the health of the workforce improved. After all, it is the ethical thing to do.

Commitment 10: "We will ensure that the victims of mental injury receive the same degree of medical care as the victims of physical injuries."

When someone is physically hurt, they will receive treatment on site and if required be transferred to a doctor or hospital. Organisations recognise they have a duty of care.

How often does this happen with a mental injury?

To show how different things can be, the Regional Engineering Manager at a major consultancy responded to news of a mental injury which occurred on his watch with:

"I was shocked to read about the impact of recent events on your mental well-being, and would strongly urge you to contact and discuss your issues with your GP, a counsellor or the Samaritans (call 116 123), which in my experience have provided excellent support"

In other words *"Your mental health is yours to maintain, not ours."* This highlights the difference between a mental health approach and a recognition of mental injury.

Organisations should therefore have contingency arrangements for the treatment of the victims of mental injury. This will obviously be different to the response to a physical injury and that is why procedures need to be developed in advance. This might involve specialist medical assistance and counselling.

And, of course, it's important that the event is logged and an investigation is launched. One of the differences between a physical injury and a mental injury is the timescale. The former will generally (but not always) be revealed instantaneously whereas the latter might only emerge over time. Having a good system of open and honest reporting can help to address this. When a person suffers a physical event, medical assistance will frequently be provided on a contingency basis, often as a check-up. If we are to be serious about mental safety, we need to make similar arrangements.

There is a growing number of organisations providing mental health first aiders in the workplace. This is good and can be utilised so long as suitable modifications are made as required. This might involve:

- Ensuring the organisation is fully committed to mental safety. After all, the aim should be prevention rather than cure.
- Ensuring the first aid training addresses mental safety adequately.

Commitment 11: "There will be no retribution against those who report mental injuries."

Some years ago, a contractor suffered a case of Prepatellar Bursitis ("Housemaids's Knee") on a North Sea platform. When he was picked up at the heliport by his employer, he was immediately berated for having lost them a £60,000 bonus they would have received for achieving a particular safety target. There are of course issues as to whether money should revolve around safety performance, but by and large things have improved with respect to safety since then. It is a given that there should be no retribution against those reporting safety events. There is also the concept of Just Culture, but that is a different matter which I will address later.

So there should be no retribution for reporting mental injuries. In our case study, when Company A had failed to do what was right and, with their verbal agreement, I raised the matter with Company B. I had to continue to pursue it. Later on Company A, as well as supporting a false allegation, threatened me with legal action for standing up for due process!

Commitment 12: "We will impose similar requirements on our contractors."

Given the nature of the modern world many members of the workforce (or those involved in the endeavour in some way) will be employed by other organisations or be self-employed. Hence, it is important to spread the care for mental safety through the supply chain. Broadly speaking, if the client cares about mental safety, the contractor will. Conversely, if the client doesn't care about mental safety not just in their own organisation but through the supply chain, the contractor may not care or may find it commercially attractive not to.

There's an analogy for this in the fashion industry. For a number of years the demand for ever-cheaper clothes grew and retailers were happy to provide them. They did this by progressively moving from one low labour cost area to another. There was little or no concern by the retailers or the consumer why the garments were so cheap. In recent years, there has been increased interest in the supply chain, driven in part by some disastrous events such as 2013 Dhaka garment factory collapse in Bangladesh.[38] There has also been a focus on the rates of pay for workers and the application of modern slavery in the supply chain. Why do I mention this? Because retailers have been forced to look more deeply into their supply chain and not just rejoice in low prices. Likewise, organisations need to care about how the staff in their contractors are being treated, especially mentally.

Every organisation should have a way of selecting and monitoring contractors and suppliers which includes health and safety as well as other factors such as commercial and technical. This will generally take various forms:

- Prior to deciding who should receive invitations to tender, there will generally be a pre-qualification (PQ) process. This is a coarse filtering stage of seeing who would identify themselves as a contender and determining if they meet a series of minimum hurdles. One of these hurdles will generally be health and safety. Mental safety should be built in at this stage by identifying if they even have a suitable policy in place.

- The next stage is the invitation to tender (ITT) when requests for detailed proposals are made. In this stage, further information is generally requested on health and safety matters. This is a great opportunity to probe their real commitment to mental safety including their track record.

- Having awarded a contract, there is the operational phase during which the delivery against a number of metrics is monitored. Audits may also be undertaken. The metrics can include one or two for mental safety. If a number of major organisations started doing this, it would send an earthquake through the supply chain. Even if it doesn't contribute to your own organisation's performance directly, it is ethical to demand that people in your supply chain are treated with respect and not exposed to the risk of mental injury.

---

[38] The Rana Plaza collapse was caused by a structural failure. The death toll was 1,134. It's thought to be the deadliest structural failure accident in modern human history and the deadliest garment factory disaster in history. The building's owners ignored warnings to avoid using it after cracks had appeared the day before. Garment workers were ordered to return the following day, and the building collapsed during the morning rush hour.

3. How do I go about integrating mental safety?

As I ponder the matter of mental safety and how it is such an overlooked area, I wonder why organisations who care about other areas of safety can ignore this one.

Organisations claim to be ethical and to stand up for what is right. And yet, in reality, all too many of them will prioritise profit or other goals unless and until influenced by other factors.

These influences could be legal, regulatory, societal or stakeholders.

It is in this way that companies have been forced to become more focused to one degree or another on process safety, personal safety, environmental issues, slavery, child labour, etc.

So how could they be influenced to adopt mental safety?

- It is already a legal responsibility in many jurisdictions. Regulators need to emphasise this and enforce it.

- Staff – as crucial stakeholders – need to demand it through their safety representatives and consultation forums.

- Shareholders – as the ultimate owners of the company to whom the executives are responsible – should insist on it.

- There needs to be more open publicity around mental safety failures.

- There could even be an award for mental safety. Perhaps one of my readers would like to sponsor one!

These are just a few initial thoughts. Now let's imagine that you have decided to implement a mental safety programme.

How would you go about it?

You might do the work internally or you might bring in a consultant.

If you do the latter, I strongly recommend that you select a consultant which has applied the principles themselves.

If you are taking on a process safety consultant, you can't expect them to have applied all the principles in their own business since they probably won't have the opportunity.

If you are taking on a personal safety consultant, you can expect them to have applied the techniques so far as the opportunities are available.

But if you are appointing a mental safety consultant, there is no excuse for them not having applied the mental safety principles in their entirety.

So, you might say: "Can you name a consultant which has applied all these principles?"

Unfortunately, I can't just now – and that speaks volumes about the world we live in – but if anyone thinks their company fits the bill, please get in touch!

Astoundingly, even consultancies that market themselves as health and safety experts (even human factors specialists) generally don't understand or apply these concepts when it comes to mental safety in the own organisation. Apart from other considerations, unless they have implemented the principles, how do they know what they are and whether they work?

Having decided on whether or not to use external assistance, you need to establish it as a project, with a project manager and a project plan.

You could start by developing a set of commitments such as the ones in this book and undertaking a survey against them to see how well you are perceived to comply with them. This will give you a gap analysis. You can also seek to identify historical lapses that have taken place. Records of staff absence might be of assistance as might the stories that your people have to tell. These stories can be used as demonstrations of where you have come from and from where you wish to improve.

Indeed you can create a storybook of *"This is where we've come from"* and *"This is our future path"*. After a period of time, the book can be revisited and rewritten.

It's important as you progress that you engage in meaningful consultation with the workforce and are ready to be "called out" for behaviour that seems to be inconsistent with the new aspirations.

You can also undertake further anonymous surveys periodically to gain continual insight into how well you are doing and whether real change is being detected.

In time, of course, your organisation's reputation should grow as an attractive place to work. Virtue can sometimes be its own reward!

4. The power of the apology

Occasionally, people do something with the possibility of causing a mental injury but then manage to snatch victory from the jaws of defeat through a well-timed apology.

More often, they dig themselves further into the entrenched position they have created.

Some years ago, one of the telegraph poles feeding our estate was demolished by a car. Obviously we lost telephone and internet access. It seemed an eternity while BT fixed it, but finally the work commenced. About 4 pm on the day the work was completed, the door bell rang. I could see it was a telephone engineer and raced to the door to give him my frustrations with both barrels. But before I could get going, he opened with the following memorable phrase "If I was you, I'd be p***ed off with how long it's taken to fix this." In just a few words, he had defused the situation.

It's not an admission of weakness to apologise but a show of inner strength!

5. Don't be dysfunctional!

Many mental injuries arise from or are compounded by organisational dysfunction.

This can be dysfunctionality within organisations or dysfunctionality between organisations – or both.

In our case study, two organisations were involved. Both proved to be internally chaotic. The correspondence within Company B obtained under GDPR showed the disbelief in those parts of the organisation who knew me about what had occurred. I was even referred to as being their "HAZOP facilitator of choice." They sought to establish an investigation but were foiled. Another part of the organisation felt it was acceptable to take the action they did and this has been supported ever since by senior management.

Likewise Company A had a mass of different people involved from at least four different offices and a complete reluctance to rock the boat with the client.

But beyond that, the contractual relationship between them led to Company A having to put to one side the ethical and professional norms that should have formed their cultural backbone.

Does your organisation have a commitment to mental safety that is so strong that there can be no scope for dysfunctionality? Furthermore, are you always – without exception – prepared to stand up for what is right? To apply the principles of ALARP[39] to mental safety?

---

[39] See Chapter 6.

CHAPTER SIX

SAFETY PRINCIPLES

I now want to move on to discuss some general safety principles that can and should be applied to mental safety.

1. The ALARP principle

We often hear people talk about things being "totally safe", although no such situation exists. As I write this book the world is in the grip of COVID-19[40] and UK schools are reopening. So often in the media we hear people talk about the necessity of the schools being totally safe before students can return. I have even heard politicians assuring the nation that they are.

The reality is that the world can never be risk-free or totally safe.

A key principle in UK health and safety legislation is that of ALARP, which stands for As Low as Reasonably Practicable, referring to the risk. An understanding of this is crucial for mental safety and indeed for life.

In deciding if something is ALARP, there are two standards that should be applied:

- Has good practice been applied?
- Is there anything that can cost-effectively be done to further reduce the risk? This latter principle was defined during the case of *Edwards vs the National Coal Board* in 1949. Mr Edwards was a miner who was killed when an underground roadway in a mine collapsed. The case concerned whether the NCB had adequately shored up the roadways in the mine. The case revolved around the use of the expression "reasonably practicable" in the Coal Mines Act 1911. In a landmark judgement, the court ruled that "Reasonably practicable is a narrower term than 'Physically possible' and implies that a computation must be made […] in which the quantum of risk is placed in one scale and the sacrifice involved in the measures necessary for averting the risk

---

[40] COVID stands for Coronavirus Infectious Disease. The 19 stands for 2019, the year of its discovery.

> (whether in time, trouble or money) is placed in the other and that, if it be shown that there is a great disproportion between them – the risk being insignificant in relation to the sacrifice – the person upon whom the obligation is imposed discharges the onus which is upon him."

Whilst this latter aspect gets much airtime, the former aspect often gets neglected but is important. Much of my career over the past twelve years has been associated with process safety. When we are evaluating whether a design is ALARP, we have to first confirm that good practice, generally as defined within industry codes and standards, has been applied. If it hasn't been, there needs to be very sound reasoning. To get clarity over this, the barrier model can help.

Where there is the possibility of a hazardous event which could lead to an undesired consequence, we ensure there are a series of barriers in place to reduce the likelihood of the ultimate consequence crystallising. We use more than one barrier because any barrier can fail to operate as planned.

So we can construct a barrier diagram as shown. We need to have sufficient barriers to reduce the mitigated likelihood of an event to an acceptable level based on the extent of the possible consequence.

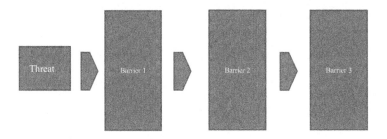

If we have a vessel that can be overpressurised, this might work as follows:

- The threat or the cause could be a valve failing open, leading to excess flow into the vessel and hence a build up in pressure.

- **Barrier 1** might be an alarm. This should be independent of the cause. This would require operator intervention. No alarm and perhaps especially its operator action is perfect.

- **Barrier 2** might be a safety instrumented system. This would consist of an independent sensor, logic solver and valve to shut off the flow into the vessel. No safety instrumented system is perfect.

- **Barrier 3** would typically be a relief valve. This may come as a surprise to many people, but relief valves aren't perfect either.

So we have a series of imperfect but independent devices, and overall the protection would be judged adequate when taking all of the chances of failure into account. There are generally accepted industry standards for the protection of systems. These can be supplemented by undertaking a HAZOP study and a Layer of Protection Analysis (LOPA). The LOPA will demonstrate that a tolerable likelihood of the event occurring has been achieved. In this case, it would typically be of the order of once per million years, depending on the number of people at risk.

Bullying

Let's see how this applies to mental safety, taking the example of bullying.

Bullying can take various forms. It can come down the management chain, it can be peer-to-peer or it can be a group bullying an individual. In this example, I am going to focus on the first type.

The first thing is to determine what the credible consequence is. Bullying can credibly lead to suicide, since there is a wealth of documented examples of this. For example, George Cheese, an apprentice mechanic at an Audi garage in Reading was bullied by his co-workers[41]. They locked him in a cage, doused him in brake fluid and set his clothes set on fire. One told him he should "hurry up and kill himself". Unfortunately, he did.

Having determined the credible consequence, we can establish a target frequency, i.e. a frequency that mustn't be exceeded for the

---

[41] The Guardian, 25 May 2017.

event. In this case, the target frequency might be set as once in 10,000 years or 10^{-4}. The frequency is achieved by a mixture of:

- Minimising the likelihood of the initiating event.
- Having sufficient barriers in place to reduce the likelihood of the event leading to a suicide.

These barriers are, in this case, the checks and balances that should detect any bullying or possibility of bullying and prevent or detect it. As with the pressure vessel example above, the barriers are not perfect and there is a risk of each of them failing. That is why we need multiple barriers, which should be as independent of each other as possible.

What type of barriers might we apply? In this case, any barriers that we define will not have the same reliability as most of the ones we use in process safety, since they will depend on people, who are notably unpredictable and unreliable, and complex interactions. Nonetheless, this may be the best that we have.

Let's identify some suitable barriers, but before we do that, I want to return to the initiating event. This must be reduced so far as possible. That depends on having suitable recruitment and training processes in place to reduce the possibility of a bullying episode. It also depends on not having undue pressure on people to deliver which can lead to mixed messages. The more work you can do to reduce the likelihood of the event, the fewer barriers you have to identify and maintain.

So having reduced the likelihood of a bullying event, we now need to establish some suitable barriers that can detect it and stop it if it occurs, to reduce the likelihood of it leading to our credible outcome of a fatality.

What might some suitable barriers be? Here are some thoughts:

- Management need to be aware what their subordinates are doing and be willing to intervene. Where the person concerned is the Chief Executive, the board need to be observant and also willing to take action. This can, of course, be difficult since people don't generally reach such elevated positions by being shy and retiring, but it is necessary.

- There can be independent helplines for people to call if bullying occurs.

- Peers can observe bullying in progress and may be able to intervene.

This can be tabulated as:

Cause: Bullying			
Potential Outcome: Suicide.			
Reduce likelihood of cause	Barrier 1	Barrier 2	Barrier 3
Recruitment. Training. No undue pressure on people to deliver.	Management observation and intervention.	Independent helplines for people to call if bullying occurs.	Peer observation and intervention.

Hannah Kirkham, 18, was attacked and humiliated by some of her colleagues at KFC in Manchester. Her mother found her collapsed on her bedroom floor on 17th December 2003. She died in hospital nine days later. The jury said she meant to kill herself by taking an overdose, was clinically depressed and this was "significantly influenced" by bullying at work. KFC said it introduced anti-bullying policies, including a confidential helpline, **following** her death. What a shame they didn't have these and other systems in place beforehand.

All of the barriers depend on people, which makes them by nature quite weak and therefore in need of continuous regeneration and reinforcement. Furthermore, barriers should so far as possible be independent and so it's important that these don't all rely on the same person taking action. It's for that reason in process safety that we will generally only take credit for one alarm because no matter how independent the alarms might be in terms of technology (they may have separate sensors, separate logic solvers and even separate annunciator systems) they will generally require the same operator to take action.

Without getting involved in the detailed mathematics, if the target frequency is to be achieved, there need to be a minimum of two and preferably three robust barriers in place in addition to the work required to reduce the likelihood of bullying in the first place. As has been demonstrated, the hurdles are incredibly high.

A challenge is to determine how robust each of those barriers really is. In process safety we have extensive inspection, maintenance and auditing systems which help us to have confidence in our defences. A relief valve, for example, isn't subject to "fit and forget". It's given regular visual examinations to ensure there is no obvious deterioration and it's tested regularly to ensure it will lift at the right pressure. And if it either fails to lift as required or lifts prematurely it is investigated. All of those things come together to help us determine what we call the probability of failure on demand.

"Now," you might say "you are using the analogy of process safety which is about stopping major accident hazards such as major fire and explosion in which many people can be killed. Mental safety is surely more analogous to occupational safety where you don't have the same confidence in barriers."

True. So let's look at occupational safety. First and foremost, the same principle applies. We look at the unmitigated consequence and use that to establish a tolerable frequency. Then we ensure we have sufficient barriers in place to ensure the situation is tolerable. Let's look at an example.

There is a stretch-wrap machine to wrap palletised loads[42]. The first task is to hypothesise how people can be hurt. Moving parts can trap fingers, hands, arms etc, causing crush injuries. Furthermore, the whole body may also get trapped between a moving pallet load and a fixed structure.

We conclude that it's credible that a serious injury could result. This tells us that we need a number of effective and independent barriers. These might be:

- Only standard palletised loads will be wrapped, obviating the use of unusual loads that might lead to imbalances, etc.
- The area around machine will be kept unobstructed at all times

---

[42] Example is based on one on the H&SE website hse.gov.uk

- The area around the machine will be indicated using fluorescent orange-red.
- Weekly checks will be performed on guarding and the condition of machine.
- Staff will be trained to use the machine correctly.
- Mechanical parts will be maintained regularly.
- Fixed guards will be fitted on moving parts
- An emergency stop button will be provided.

You will notice that there are more barriers here than for the process safety event above. That might be surprising but can be explained by the following:

1. With occupational safety we are more dependent on people who are less dependable than instrumentation.

2. There is as mentioned previously a separate aspect to ALARP, i.e. is there anything that can cost-effectively be done to further reduce the risk? In theory this means identifying additional safeguards and for each one to calculate the incremental whole-life cost and the incremental benefit. The incremental benefit (the value of the theoretical fatality or serious injury averted x the incremental reduction in its likelihood) is translated into money. This will come as a surprise to many people. How often do we hear the expressions *"you can't put a price on a human life"* or *"you can't put a price on safety"*? Well, we can and we do, because that allows us how to best, as a society, allocate finite resources. When we are dealing with process safety the incremental expenditures are relatively high, generally involving new hardware which has to be bought, inspected and maintained. With occupational safety the incremental expenditures are often quite modest: a new procedure or an amendment to a training course, for example, so it is reasonable to do more things. Typical costs per injury type are generally publicised in the various regulatory regimes. In the UK they can be found the H&SE website. In round number terms the cost of a human life is assessed as being about £1.3 million at the time of writing.

Other causes of mental injury may be assessed as follows:

Cause: Allegations			
Potential Outcome: Where a **false** allegation is made, it can lead to mental injury.			
Reduce likelihood of cause	**Barrier 1**	**Barrier 2**	**Barrier 3**
Training. Culture of positive behaviours and positive culture.	Initial investigation and validation before being progressed.	Further investigation interviewing the person the allegation concerns.	

Cause: Harassment			
Potential Outcome: Mental injury.			
Reduce likelihood of cause	**Barrier 1**	**Barrier 2**	**Barrier 3**
Policy statement communication. Training.	Management observation and intervention.	Independent helplines for people to call if harassment occurs.	Peer observation and intervention.

2. HR or safety?

"Surely much of this is in hand through the human resource function?" I hear some people saying.

It's certainly true that the causes of mental injury are often seen to be the responsibility of HR. The CIPD (Chartered Institute of Personnel and Development) has produced guidance notes on many of these aspects.[43] These guidance notes lay out the legal framework. Bullying, for example, is addressed as follows:

> "The legal position on bullying is more complex [than harassment] as there's no single piece of legislation which

---

[43] See for example "Harassment and bullying at work", CIPD, 30 Jun 2020

deals with workplace bullying. In the UK, bullying may be covered by:

- The Equality Act 2010, if it is linked to a protected characteristic.
- The Employment Rights Act 1996, especially the 'detriment' provisions.
- Claims for breach of an express or implied term of the employment contract – for example, breach of the implied term to take care of employees' safety or provide reasonable support to ensure they can work without harassment and disruption by fellow workers.
- Criminal or civil provisions under the Protection from Harassment Act 1998.

Bullying might also be covered by a myriad of other legal principles and laws, for example:

- The common law obligation for an employer to take care of workers' safety.
- Personal injury protection involving the duty to take care of workers arising out of the law of Tort.
- Health and Safety at work etc Act 1974.
- Public Order Act 1986.
- Trade Union and Labour Relations (Consolidation) Act 1992 – dealing with special types of intimidation.
- Criminal Justice and Public Order Act 1994.
- Protection for whistleblowers under the Public Interest Disclosure Act 1998.
- Human Rights Act 1998."

The purpose of this book is not to dismiss this but to complement what has been and is being done by the HR profession with a safety insight, especially with regard to the actual harm that can be done to individuals. You'll note that the CIPD extract above refers to the Health and Safety at work etc Act 1974, recognising the safety implications.

What is clear is that Boards of organisations need to focus on mental safety in the same way they care about other aspects of safety. A board level director should have an explicit remit for mental safety across the organisation. Who this is (HR, safety or other) matters less than their familiarity with the subject matter and with safety. They need to ensure there is a plan for implementing and monitoring mental safety consistent with other safety activities. A relevant Board committee should also have it in their remit.

3.   The importance of warning signs

A colleague once said to me "The absence of bad news can itself be bad news." He had been investigating an event on an offshore platform where an accumulator had been overpressurised during maintenance and exploded leading to a technician losing several fingers. When he was looking into this, he found that all appeared to be well on the installation prior to this event. As he looked deeper, though, he discovered that there wasn't sufficient identification of straws in the wind that with a bit of insight might have warned of a looming issue, if not this one in particular. There can sometimes be excessive complacency.

Many organisations have ways of monitoring their safety culture and data for potential issues, but few – if any – have a way of scanning for potential mental safety issues. This is hardly surprising since few – if any – have a real concept of mental safety.

What might these warning signs look like?

- Top of the pile is any sense of **corporate complacency on the one hand** ("we have a real concern for mental safety") **or a complete absence of awareness of mental safety on the other**. It's also not adequate to assert that it's all covered under the mental health agenda because those agendas, although highly beneficial, have proved to be inadequate on their own.

- Then there is an **aggressive culture in which ends justify means**. This is all too common. Certain sectors are famous (perhaps infamous) for this. Investment banking comes to mind. Actually, scrub the word "investment" there. Fred Goodwin was one of the architects of the financial crisis in the UK in 2008. He had become CEO of Royal Bank of Scotland in 2001 and led a programme of dramatic expansion which ended in disaster not just for RBS but for the nation as a £45.5 billion bail out was required. Goodwin was famous for his aggressiveness not just in business expansion but for his dealings with people. His colleagues reported that 'He manufactured fear'; 'Fred was your classic bully.'[44] The Board should never have appointed him since they knew his character traits before they did. His legacy was so bad that RBS has now rebranded itself as Natwest, which had been taken over by RBS in 2000.

- **Indications of fear or nervousness in the workforce**. Tim Kuppler has identified the following indicators of fear in the workforce[45]:

  - Bad behaviour isn't visibly confronted.
  - Compensation, incentives and/or promotions are based on results, not results AND behaviour.
  - "Explosions" are evident periodically from one or more top leaders.
  - Pre-meetings are the norm.
  - Communication is poor or one-way.
  - Email is used to cover your rear or is not proactively used.
  - A general lack of clarity and alignment about managing work.
  - Values and expected behaviours are not specifically defined and reinforced.

- **Patterns of behaviour in particular individuals**. When a mental safety event occurs, it should scarcely ever come as a surprise. A bully is generally a consistent bully. A person who belittles subordinates or other people normally makes a practice of it. This isn't to say that they bully or belittle everyone; they often have favourite victims, frequently those who are unable to adequately stand up to it. But there should generally be evidence if people are alert to it or care about it. The Jockey Club is the UK's largest commercial horse racing organisation. Until 2006 it was responsible for the governance and regulation of British horseracing. It owns fifteen racecourses, including Aintree, Cheltenham, Epsom

---

[44] Iain Martin, Making It Happen: Fred Goodwin, RBS and the men who blew up the British economy, Simon & Schuster, 2014,
[45] The 8 Clear Signs of a Workplace Culture of Fear, Tim Kuppler, TLNT.com, 14 November 2013.

Downs and both the Rowley Mile and July Course in Newmarket. It also owns the National Stud and the property and land management company, Jockey Club Estates. In July 2019 it announced with great excitement that Delia Bushell had been appointed Group Chief Executive. In August 2020 she was forced to resign after complaints were made about her. An independent barrister, Jack Mitchell, is asserted to have found evidence to support a number of the allegations of misconduct against her – including bullying, racist comments and sharing offensive materials. It would be interesting to know whether, as well as inquiring into the allegations, an investigation was undertaken into whether this was a pattern of behaviour which could reasonably have been identified before she was appointed. But at least the Jockey Club undertook an investigation into the allegations before taking action. Not everyone is afforded this courtesy. It should be noted that Bushell is disputing the findings.

- **Staff feedback**. Feedback from the workforce is important. This can be in the instant, i.e. when some unacceptable behaviour takes place, or through the appraisal system, or through an anonymous reporting system. Feedback can be sought specifically on the propensity of people to engage in activity which could lead to mental injury such as bullying, belittlement, etc. Feedback should be sought from contractors as well as staff and taken seriously. Staff feedback can be a barrier as well as a warning sign and thus must be taken very seriously.

- **Data**. There is a wide range of data that can be used as warning signs of potential system failure such as:

  o Staff turnover levels by department
  o Absence levels
  o Frequency and duration of absences
  o Analyses of events such as grievance and discipline

Staff turnover and absences should be analysed to determine first of all whether they could conceivably be work-related in whole or in part. It's clearly none of our business to poke our noses into people's private lives, but if there's a hint of the absence being work-related it should be investigated as we have discussed previously to identify where the system can be tightened up.

So organisations need to develop means of identifying mental safety warning signs in their organisation in the same way they do for other safety matters.

To see why this is important, I draw attention to the accident triangle as first defined by Herbert Heinrich[46] and refined by Frank Bird.

Although some doubts have been placed on the nature of the research he undertook,[47] Heinrich's work is still frequently quoted and the principles are logically reasonable. Heinrich was an Assistant Superintendent of the Engineering and Inspection Division of Travelers Insurance Company and wanted to reduce the number of serious industrial accidents. He reviewed over 75,000 accident reports from his company's files and elsewhere. From this data he proposed a relationship that for each major injury accident there would be 29 minor injury accidents and 300 no-injury accidents. He concluded that by reducing the number of minor accidents industrial companies would see a correlating fall in the number of major accidents.

The relationship is often shown as a triangle or pyramid. Heinrich also suggested that 88% of all accidents were caused by a human decision to carry out an unsafe act.

In 1966 Frank Bird amended the triangle to show a ratio of one serious injury accident to 10 minor injury (first aid only) accidents, to 30 damage causing accidents, to 600 near misses.[48] He showed a relationship between the number of reported near misses and the number of major accidents and claimed that the majority of accidents could be predicted and prevented by an appropriate intervention.

The importance of this is not so much the numbers but the principle. By identifying and analysing low level events, worse ones can be averted. In mental safety, a suicide (which will be at the top of the triangle) may be averted by identifying warning signs. Along the

---

[46] Industrial Accident Prevention: A Scientific Approach, William Heinrich

[47] Examining the Foundation, Ashley Johnson, Safety and Health, October 2011

[48] Damage Control, Frank Bird, 1966

way, we avoid less serious mental safety outcomes, but also reduce staff absences, with the associated business benefits.

Although the main thrust of this book is about avoiding inflicting mental injury on people, it's worth mentioning that approximately 20% of people who have died by suicide have a history of self harm.[49]

4. The right to be heard

A well-known cause of mental injury is a feeling of not being heard. Of being out of control of your destiny. Of having things done to you. Of being abused. Of being deprived of your human rights. Of being up against a machine against which you are powerless as the initial event is frequently followed by obfuscation, denial and cover-up.

There is such a thing as natural justice. Article 10 of the United Nations Declaration of Human Rights codified this as; *"Everyone is entitled in full equality to a fair and public hearing by an independent and impartial tribunal, in the determination of his rights and obligations and of any criminal charge against him."*

The Bible tells us: *"One witness is not enough to convict anyone accused of any crime or offense they may have committed. A matter must be established by the testimony of two or three witnesses."* (Deuteronomy 19:15).

And yet too often people are still condemned without being given a fair hearing.

This, of course, occurred in our case study when Companies A and B both chose to go into writing with untruths, despite each of them having been advised in advance that they were wrong. The Associate Director at Company A even uttered the damning words: "I'm not interested [in due process], only our relationship with Company B".

5. Discipline and Just Culture

There have to be consequences for failure to behave properly.

---

[49] Foster T, Gillespie K, McClelland R. Mental disorders and suicide in Northern Ireland. Br J Psychiatry 1997;170:447-52.

We apply this in safety. Some organisations will lash out randomly if there is an incident and even dismiss people involved without consideration. This can lead to cover ups and an atmosphere of fear.

At the other end of the spectrum there is the so called "no blame" culture where promises are made of no retaliation to encourage a frank engagement with the investigation process.

In the middle is the "Just Culture". Just Culture works on the premise that mistakes leading to accidents are the result of corporate or systems failures rather than just the product of human error. It therefore tries to avoid questions like "who is responsible?" or "who gets the sack?" and instead ask "what went wrong?" That isn't to say that there are no repercussions. Areas where people made errors are still identified and some action will be taken, especially where people have wilfully done the wrong thing, but it is seen to be just.

A Just Culture is frequently seen to be part of an effective safety culture.

On 23rd March 2005 there was a devastating explosion at bp's Texas City plant which killed fifteen people. It resulted from the overfilling of a distillation column on the isomerisation unit which led to the lifting of relief valves and the release of volatile hydrocarbon liquids from an atmospheric vent. This resulted in a large vapour cloud and then an explosion and fire. The bp report was issued on 12th March 2005.[50] This was accompanied by disciplinary action against a number of operational staff. However given that the failings were due as much to management failings as operational error and perhaps more, it was surprising that no immediate action was taken at more senior levels. This smacked of the old-school kneejerk response. It was only in February 2007 that bp reported on the accountability of senior bp staff and it was initially kept confidential.[51] The report was created by a team of bp executives and legal counsel and developed four accountability tiers, with Tier 1 representing the highest level of accountability. They examined the accountability of a number of managers but concluded that only four individuals fell into Tier 1:

- Mike Hoffman, vice president, refining and marketing.
- Pat Gower, regional vice president, U.S. refining.

[50] Isomerization Unit Explosion Interim Report Texas City, Texas, USA. bp.
[51] Management Accountability Project, bp, February 2007.

- Don Parus, Texas City refinery manager.
- Willie Willis, manufacturing delivery leader for the Texas City West Plant and manager of the isomerization unit, where the blast occurred.

While Hoffman, Gower and Parus held bp Group leadership posts and Willis was a middle-level manager, the report justified Willis' inclusion by noting that Willis was being groomed as "a potential future refinery manager and group leader."

The team concluded that the four men "failed to perform their management accountabilities in significant ways." They called on bp to "seek ways to conclude their employment relationships on fair and just terms, in a timely manner."

In a separate report, the team placed John Manzoni, chief executive of bp's refining and marketing segment, in Tier 2, but stopped short of calling for Manzoni's termination. They said:

> *"Process safety did not have the same priority, at least, as commercial issues for [Manzoni], and there were important performance gaps from a management accountability perspective concerning his actions (or inactions)," the team wrote. " ... While it is evident that this did not contribute to the fundamental root causes for the [isomerization unit] disaster, it is not simply hindsight to suggest that John should have taken more steps to consider and mitigate the risks long before this disaster occurred."*

There is no documented evidence of any action being taken against Manzoni and he moved on to become head of Talisman Energy. He then became chief executive of the UK civil service and the Cabinet Office Permanent Secretary from 2014 to 2020. He was appointed Knight Commander of the Order of the Bath (KCB) in the 2020 New Year Honours for public service.

Although bp's approach to Just Culture over Texas City was seen to be somewhat patchy, it was at least undertaken, especially at senior levels. Just Culture should be applied at all relevant levels to mental safety events as well as process safety and personal safety. It should be assessing behaviour against safety standards and not just employment (HR) standards.

6. Mental Safety Culture

So let's talk about safety culture and how this can evolve into a mental safety culture.

40 years ago – about the time I graduated – no one talked about safety culture.

On 25th April 1986, routine maintenance was scheduled at reactor number 4 at the Chernobyl nuclear plant in Ukraine. It was intended to use the downtime to test whether the reactor could still be cooled if the plant lost power. During the test, workers violated safety protocols and power surged inside the plant. Despite attempts to shut down the reactor entirely, another power surge caused a chain reaction of explosions. Finally, the nuclear core itself was exposed, discharging radioactive material into the atmosphere. The use of the expression "safety culture" is generally recognised to have emerged in the International Atomic Energy Agency's initial report into the disaster[52].   Cultural defects have emerged in almost every major accident hazard since.

Safety culture has been defined by the CBI as *"the way we do things around here"*[53].

The UK Health & Safety Executive's Advisory Committee on the Safety of Nuclear Installations produced a definition [54] as follows:

'The safety culture of an organisation is the product of individual and group values, attitudes, perceptions, competencies, and patterns of behaviour that determine the commitment to, and the style and proficiency of, an organisation's health and safety management'.

'Organisations with a positive safety culture are characterised by communications founded on mutual trust, by shared perceptions of

---

[52] INSAG, Summary Report on the Post-Accident Review Meeting on the Chernobyl Accident, published by the IAEA as Safety Series No.75-INSAG-l, 1986.
[53] Confederation of British Industry (CBI) Report, 1990. Developing a Safety Culture- Business for Safety.
[54] Health and Safety Commission (HSC). 1993. ACSNI Study Group on Human Factors. 3rd Report: Organising for Safety. (London: HMSO).

the importance of safety and by confidence in the efficacy of preventive measures'.

However you define it, every organisation has a safety culture. These cultures could be positioned on a spectrum with "anything will do" at one end and "mature" at the other. Some organisations have worked hard to develop, implement and audit their cultures. Others haven't bothered. What is certain, though, is that very few organisations have considered mental safety as an important part of their culture. They may have a commitment to mental health but that is insufficient.

What I advocate is not that mental safety is prioritised but that the corporate safety culture – in whatever state of development – includes mental safety. If the safety culture needs to improve, then let mental safety improve alongside personal safety and process safety.

According to the UK H&SE, symptoms of **poor** cultural factors can include[55]:

- Widespread, routine procedural violations;
- Failure to comply with the company's own safety management system (although either of these can also be due to poor procedure design);
- Management decisions that appear consistently to put production or cost before safety.

On the other hand, the UK H&SE has identified key aspects of an **effective** culture as including:[56]

- **Management commitment**: this commitment produces higher levels of motivation and concern for health and safety throughout the organisation. It is indicated by the proportion of resources (time, money and people) and support allocated to health and safety management and by the status given to health and safety versus production, cost etc. The active involvement of senior management in the health and safety system is very important.

- **Visible management**: Managers need to be seen to lead by example when it comes to health and safety. Good managers

---

[55] H&SE, Common topic 4: Safety culture
[56] H&SE, Common topic 4: Safety culture

---

appear regularly on the 'shop floor', talk about health and safety and visibly demonstrate their commitment by their actions – such as stopping production to resolve issues. It is important that management is perceived as sincerely committed to safety. If not, employees will generally assume that they are expected to put commercial interests first, and safety initiatives or programmes will be undermined by cynicism.

- **Good communications** between all levels of employee: in a positive culture questions about health and safety should be part of everyday work conversations. Management should listen actively to what they are being told by employees, and take what they hear seriously.

- Active **employee participation** in safety is important, to build ownership of safety at all levels and exploit the unique knowledge that employees have of their own work. This can include active involvement in workshops, risk assessments, plant design etc. In companies with a good culture, you will find the story from employees and management being consistent, and safety is seen as a joint exercise.

All of this could and should be applied to mental safety. Imagine how different the world would be if there was:

- **Management commitment to mental safety**: the commitment of management produces higher levels of motivation and concern for mental safety throughout the organisation. It is indicated by the proportion of resources (time, money and people) and support allocated to mental safety and by the status given to mental safety versus production, cost etc. There is active involvement of senior management in mental safety.

- **Visible management**: Managers are seen to lead by example in mental safety. Managers appear regularly on the 'shop floor', talk about mental safety and visibly demonstrate their commitment by their actions. Management is perceived as sincerely committed to mental safety. Employees must not assume they are expected to put commercial interests first. Mental Safety isn't undermined by cynicism.

- **Good communications between all levels of employee (and contractors)**: Questions about mental safety are part of everyday work conversations. Management listen actively to what they are being told by employees and contractors, and take what they hear seriously.

- Active **employee participation** in mental safety is important and builds ownership of mental safety at all levels and exploits the unique knowledge that the workforce have of their own work. This can include active involvement in workshops, risk assessments, etc. You find the story from the workforce and management to be consistent, and mental safety is seen as a joint exercise.

7. Audits

Responsible organisations audit the application of their health, safety and environmental systems. This will frequently take the form of ongoing self-audit or self-assessment, supplemented by periodic external audits.

Furthermore, the regulators may also undertake audits.

It's fair to say that similar arrangements are rarely if ever in place for mental safety.

An audit programme is primarily designed to review how the application compares with the corporate standard, legislation, etc. This, of course, requires there to be a standard. Hence, the organisation needs to define first of all what it stands for by developing a series of standards for mental safety. These might be discrete standards or form part of other health and safety standards but the requirements for protecting mental safety need to be clearly identifiable.

Having defined the standards, an audit programme can be established. This will often take the form of:

- A continuous programme of self-audit in which the standards are reviewed by the operating teams on a regular basis, perhaps one standard per month.

- A review on a risk-weighted basis performed by a team external to the entity being audited. Typically, this might be performed once every three years but more frequently if there are significant concerns.

When I discussed the barrier model, I noted that the barriers can be weak when applied to mental safety since they rely so much on human factors. The audit programme should focus on ensuring the robustness and reliability of the barriers and of those features that reduce the likelihood of the event.

Let's look at the example of bullying:

Cause: Bullying			
Potential Outcome: Suicide			
Reduce likelihood of cause	Barrier 1	Barrier 2	Barrier 3
Recruitment. Training. No undue pressure on people to deliver.	Management observation and intervention	Independent helplines for people to call if bullying occurs.	Peer observation and intervention.

The audit programme might look at how effective:

- the recruitment system is to screen candidates;
- the training is with respect to the mental impact of bullying;
- the management culture is to avoid excessive pressure to deliver;
- the management observation systems are;
- the helplines and follow-up are; and
- the peer observation and intervention systems are.

The organisation needs to be prepared to accept the audit findings and implement them. Unfortunately, all too often people will push back against audits and criticise the auditors. This is a particular risk when dealing with ambitious, driven and forceful people whose attitude and approach might be criticised in the audit.

In order to gain backing for the audit, a terms of reference (TOR) should be prepared and authorised at a senior level in the organisation, preferably by the head of the entity being audited. This would be the Board Chair if it is being performed at a corporate level.

Audit teams need to have the right skills. For mental safety this will typically include:

- A team leader who should be an experienced auditor.
- At least one subject matter (mental safety) expert.
- Other experienced auditors are required.

Audit recommendations should be clear, standalone and risk based, for example: "The team identified that absences due to stress are not being investigated. One or more of these events may relate to mental safety issues. If not investigated, there is a risk of further serious mental injuries. The team therefore recommends that a system be developed to formally undertake investigations into all absences to identify any mental safety issues."

8.   Management of change

Organisations should have a management of change system. This is an important part of behaving both responsibly and legally in terms of managing risk.

Change takes various forms, including:

- Technical change to process plant or equipment.
- Changes to procedures.
- Organisational change.

It sounds obvious but the starting point should be to recognise that a change is about to take place. Unfortunately this isn't in the DNA of many – perhaps most – organisations.

When I worked in the North Sea oil industry, I was on a platform conducting a health, safety and environmental audit. As I strolled across the top deck of the installation I noticed some diesel generators. I proceeded to the morning management meeting which I was attending as part of the audit. At the end of it I asked a simple question: "Could I see the management of change process used for the generators?" I was advised that it wasn't necessary since they were only there temporarily. I pointed out to them that the Management of Change (MOC) system had to be applied to temporary as well as permanent change. I then said "In any case, they don't look very temporary to me: you've welded them to the deck!"

Hazards don't go away just because it's a temporary change.

This was over 25 years ago and yet putting technical change through an MOC system is still not automatic in many organisations. Less so with procedural change and even less so with organisational change.

Organisational change in particular can impact the workforce mentally. For that reason, it's important that organisational change is carefully managed through an MOC system.

By way of context, a study was undertaken into a suicide epidemic in France.[57] This looked at letters written by individuals in 82 suicide cases across three companies during the period 2005-2015. In each company, there was a peak of suicides at times of restructuring, when new management policies were being introduced either to increase workloads through raised production targets or to cut company costs by shedding jobs. In most of these letters, employees blame work or their experiences of work as the cause of their self- killing.

What are the characteristics of a good MOC system? It's about properly assessing and implementing the change.

Change starts with an idea, for example "why don't we combine two departments?" Many organisations might just jump in and effect the change, focused on the clear business and financial benefits. This will often be done with no clear plan for the wellbeing of the staff or appreciation of the risks for them, giving the leader of the new department carte blanche to do whatever is required. The business benefits may well accrue but at the risk of damaging the mental safety of staff and contractors. Often the lack of detailed planning will enhance the pressure on people as the leadership become more demanding about meeting the targets. The result may be announced

---

[57] Suicidal work: Work-related suicides are uncounted, Sarah Waters, Hazards online special report, March 2017.

as a successful transition yielding cost savings, better positioning the organisation for the future and so on. Management bonuses could result with smiling faces all around. Happy days. However, how has this been achieved? Quite possibly at the cost of at least one serious mental injury.

It's for this reason that organisational change must be subjected to control. This enables, amongst other things:

- The proper evaluation of the benefits and the costs.
- A plan to be developed.
- The risks to be evaluated and actions developed.
- Those actions to be integrated into the plan.
- Proper close out of actions.
- Authorisation at key points in the schedule.

What might be the significance of this for mental safety? Here is what a few lines might look like in the evaluation.

Aspect	Typical Issue	Possible actions
Benefits and costs	Has any consideration been taken of the mental safety costs in the light not just of the change but the overall environment?	It may be concluded that the change should be deferred because there is quite simply too much going on.
Plan	Has the plan considered the new or amended roles of people and the skills required?	Ensure the roles And responsibilities are properly defined and that appropriate training has been organised.
Risks and actions	Will people be overloaded in the early days of their new roles?	Consider phasing manpower changes to ensure a realistic workload for the new team.

It's important to have "gates" in the process where the change gets formally approved for transition to the next stage based on the actions taken in the current stage and the plans (including the risk management) into the next stage. These sign-offs should not be made glibly.

The worst possible MOC system is one where the paperwork is completed after the change has been made to meet corporate or legislative requirements. It might be hard to imagine it occurring but it's not unusual. For example, on 13th June 2013 there was a catastrophic explosion and fire at the Williams Geismar olefins[58] plant in Geismar, Louisiana. The subsequent investigation by the US Chemical Safety and Hazard Investigation Board (Generally referred to as the Chemical Safety Board or CSB) showed the MOC paperwork had been completed after installation of the valve the closure of which led to the explosion.[59]

When undertaking MOC assessments, there is generally a list of requirements and guidance notes. These should include the protection of mental safety – but how often do they fully?

---

[58] Olefins, also called alkenes, are organic compounds made up of hydrogen and carbon that contain one or more pairs of carbon atoms linked by a double bond. The simplest ones are ethylene (C_2H_4) and propylene (C_3H_6). They are used to manufacture many chemicals including polythene (which is polyethylene) and polypropylene.
[59] The CSB have made a video of the disaster called "Blocked In". It's available on the CSB website (CSB.gov) and YouTube (https://www.youtube.com/watch?v=Z1KaykPaF8M)

CHAPTER SEVEN

OTHER CONSIDERATIONS

I now want to briefly mention some other matters.

1. Professionals need to act professionally and ethically

Most if not all professions emphasise the importance of professional and ethical conduct. Unfortunately, many professionals interpret this as obviously not applying to the way they deal with people or matters outside what they regard as being their strict professional remit.

What would you think of a person who:

- Will check technical information but be willing to take an allegation against a person at face value?
- Will undertake a reorganisation which considers the financial risks in great detail but not consider the impact on mental safety?
- Will rigidly apply risk assessment when physical safety is at risk but fail to address the impact on mental safety?

Or a health board that will make many of its staff ill through bullying whilst promoting suicide prevention?

It's time for professionals to act professionally and ethically. It's also time for professional organisations (such as engineering institutions) to review whether they adequately care about these matters. Ironically, the Executive Vice President at Company A who thought it was OK to take an allegation at face value is a fellow and a trustee of the Royal Academy of Engineering.

2. The gig economy

The world of work has always been divided between company employees, sub-contractors and the self-employed. However, this has become more marked in recent years, so much so that we now hear of the "gig economy". The phrase was coined at the height of the 2008-9 financial crisis, when the unemployed made a living by "gigging" or working in several part time jobs whenever they could. The phrase has stuck and has been described as "a labour market characterised by the prevalence of short-term contracts or freelance work, as opposed to permanent jobs"[60].

Given that organisations' commitment to mental safety is generally weak and even weaker or non-existent when it comes to non-employees, this implies that more people are exposed to the risk of mental injury.

With the rise of the internet there has been a substantial increase in goods being delivered to households by van. These are frequently delivered by self-employed drivers working for delivery companies in the gig economy.

Research by University College London into the safety of gig economy drivers and riders[61] found that "The pressures that come with being a self-employed courier or taxi driver may significantly increase the risk of being involved in a collision."

The participants included self-employed couriers who delivered parcels and food, and self-employed taxi drivers who received their jobs via apps.

The majority (63%) of those surveyed weren't provided with safety training on managing risks on the road. 65% said that they weren't given any safety equipment such as a high visibility vest and over 70% resorted to providing their own.

42% of drivers and riders reported that their vehicle had been damaged as a result of a collision while working, with a further one in ten reporting that someone had been injured. 8% reported that they themselves had been injured, with 2% saying someone else had been injured.

"Our findings highlight that the emergence and rise in the popularity of gig work for couriers could lead to an increase in risk factors affecting the health and safety of people who work in the gig economy and other road users," explained the co-author. "As more workers enter the economy and competition rises, the number of hours they

---

[60] Reference not available.
[61] The emerging issues for management of occupational road risk in a changing economy: A survey of gig economy drivers, riders and their managers, Nicola Christie and Heather Ward, UCL Centre for Transport Studies, August 2018.

need to work and distances they must travel to earn a stable income both increase. We know this is an issue but don't know exactly how far it extends as not all companies need to report the number of self-employed couriers they use to the government."

As people are exposed to basic health and safety risks such as this, what chance is there of their mental safety being protected?

These drivers and riders are mainly men, who are most at risk from suicide – albeit, as we have seen, not from the underlying issues. If we are going to reduce the suicide rate, we need to work harder on mental safety.

3.   All accidents are preventable?

A common expression is "we believe that all accidents are preventable". Obviously no organisation can say the opposite!

But just how deeply does this extend to mental safety?

Let's take some examples. Company B says on its website:

> **Why it matters**
> Safety is a core value and creating a safe and healthy workplace is our top priority, involving everyone at [Company B]. Improving safety also makes us a more efficient business.
>
> **What we value**
> Cause no accidents, no harm to people and no damage to the environment.
>
> **Our approach**
> We focus on process safety, personal safety, health and wellbeing, and security:
>
> - We understand that even the best processes can have weaknesses that may lead to accidents, so we take steps to design these out.
> - We focus on preventing incidents – reacting swiftly and effectively if they happen.
> - We learn from every incident.

None of this seemed to be applicable, however, in our case study. Perhaps in referring to safety, and health and wellbeing, mental safety is excluded.

George Orwell wrote "Animal Farm" in 1943 and 1944. After considerable difficulties in finding a publisher, since the USSR[62] was an ally, it was finally published in 1945. The book is an allegory in which the animals at Manor Farm rebel against the farmer to create an ideal society. However, in the end the pigs take over and start co-operating with the humans. When the revolution starts, a set of commandments is created as follows:

- Whatever goes upon two legs is an enemy.
- Whatever goes upon four legs, or has wings, is a friend.
- No animal shall wear clothes.
- No animal shall sleep in a bed.
- No animal shall drink alcohol.
- No animal shall kill any other animal.
- All animals are equal.

At the end of the book, the commandments have been changed to:

- Four legs good, two legs better.
- No animal shall sleep in a bed with sheets.
- No animal shall drink alcohol to excess.
- No animal shall kill any other animal without cause.
- All animals are equal, but some are more equal than others.

Likewise, one could reconstruct the Company B website (and that of many other organisations) to replace safety with *safety, except mental safety* or even *mental safety, especially of contractors.*

Is the word "mental" silent when you think of "safety" and even more so when you think of "contractor safety"?

4. Mental injury as abuse

I was born in 1955. It's amazing how much abuse was occurring as I was growing up which I and most other people were totally unaware of. Admittedly, schools engaged in caning which is now banned, but up and down the country (and worldwide) there was physical and sexual abuse. There was abuse in churches, in schools, in football clubs, in gymnastics, in the Scouts and in many other places.

---

[62] "Animal Farm" is political satire about the USSR.

Frequently, the abuse was known about and covered up, perhaps most famously and extensively in the Catholic church[63], where wayward priests were frequently simply moved in the hope of avoiding scandal. Scandal descended nonetheless, albeit it delayed and having permitted further abuse to take place in the meantime. Abuse wasn't just occurring in the Catholic church. The Independent Enquiry into Sexual Abuse published a report into the Church of England in 2020.[64]

As well as being a form of physical damage, mental injury is also a form of abuse, which needs to be highlighted and stamped out in the same way as these other forms of abuse.

What do I mean by this? Abuse is "unfair, cruel, or violent treatment of someone".[65] That is certainly what it feels like when you have been the victim of a mental injury. Furthermore, whereas you aren't generally a habitual physical injurer of someone at work or elsewhere, you can be a serial mental abuser, since many of the methods of causing mental injury lend themselves to repetition. Of course, the abuser often isn't seeking to cause permanent damage and perhaps has no conception that it could occur, but that has never been an acceptable excuse and is even less so as medical science develops.

Sometimes people abuse through what is perceived to be necessity. For example, an unusual situation might have arisen and in order to get it sorted a manager might put undue pressure on people.

On the other hand, the manager might be a person who always overpressurises people. They might do this for a number of reasons. They might be poor at planning, always doing things at the last moment, and hence creating an eternal sense of panic which creates pressure. Alternatively, they might love the power they have which allows them to act in this way. Or they may even derive a kind of sadistic pleasure from it.

Jens Rasmussen, a Danish professor for system safety and human factors, developed a framework for human factors called the SRK ("Skills-Rules-Knowledge") model[66] which talks about violations as

---

[63] As depicted in the 2015 movie "Spotlight".
[64] The Anglican Church - Safeguarding in the Church of England and the Church in Wales - Investigation Report, 6th October 2020.
[65] Oxford Dictionary.
[66] Refer to "Reducing error and influencing behaviour", HSG48 (Second edition) Published 1999, UK Health and Safety Executive.

being routine, situational or exceptional. The manager who rarely puts excessive pressure on people might be classified as doing it under exceptional circumstances. The manager who always puts excessive pressure on people might be classified as doing it routinely. Then there might be a manager somewhere in between who might be classified as doing it situationally.

However, if people get away with it once or twice, they might do it more frequently, especially if they get rewarded for what they have apparently achieved.

5. It's a woke world

It's difficult to read a newspaper these days without coming across the word "woke".

"Woke" used to mean to awake after sleep.

However, "By the mid-20th century woke had been extended figuratively to refer to being 'aware' or 'well informed' in a political or cultural sense……. In the past decade, that meaning [of woke] has been catapulted into mainstream use with a particular nuance of 'alert to racial or social discrimination and injustice', popularised through the lyrics of the 2008 song Master Teacher by Erykah Badu, in which the words 'I stay woke' serve as a refrain, and more recently through its association with the Black Lives Matter movement, especially on social media"[67]

This is widely demonstrated by people taking offence on behalf of others, who quite often are not offended. In our case study, the employee from Company B declared that offence had been caused to other people when it hadn't. Howzat[68] for woke?

There is nothing wrong with being socially and culturally aware. A lack of this has been the cause of many problems (slavery, sexism, class discrimination, etc.) in the past. Whilst we must encourage staff to report what they perceive to be inappropriate or offensive behaviour it is vital that what is reported is investigated and not taken

---

[67] Oxford English Dictionary.
[68] Howzat (for "How's that?") is a cry used by cricketers when appealing to the umpire for a wicket.

at face value. If this isn't done, it can become the cause of problems in itself.

As I have described, in other forms of safety we talk of the cause-consequence model. We then apply safeguards to reduce the likelihood of the consequence occurring to a tolerable level. However, we also have to consider whether a safeguard can of itself be the cause of another hazardous event. For example, a vessel may be protected against overpressurisation by a relief valve. When we do a HAZOP on the system, we take account of the relief valve as a safeguard against excess pressure but also consider what happens if the relief valve opens in error or allows leakage. If the valve relieves to atmosphere, it may cause a toxic or flammable cloud. If it relieves into a closed system leading to a vent or flare, it may lead to blockage, corrosion or downstream slugging effects. We need to treat those as being other potentially hazardous events and ensure they are likewise mitigated.

Wokeness is intended to be a protection against unfairness and can be thought of as a kind of safeguard. As such, when improperly applied, it can also be an initiator of other unfairness. So, when developing an approach to mental safety, be sure that you help people to understand that being woke is not a license to offend in itself. People cannot in a work situation be the final arbiters of what is appropriate and be allowed to brand people as racist or sexist based purely on their (imperfect) insight. It needs to be controlled and exercised responsibly. This is yet another reason why allegations mustn't be taken at face value. Random wokeness can be the cause of mental injury. Don't be a Rogue Woke. And don't allow other people to be either.

6. Be strong

I am an active user of LinkedIn. There are many posts that tell us to "be mentally strong" and "be resilient". There are even courses in it on LinkedIn with titles such as:

- Building Resilience.
- Enhancing Resilience.
- Sheryl Sandberg and Adam Grant on Option B: Building Resilience.
- Developing Resilience and Grit.

And many, many more. If you're interested in them, you know where to look!

Resilience is important, of course, and had I been more resilient I might have shrugged off what happened to me. That would undoubtedly have saved me from considerable pain but at the same time perhaps my lack of resilience has provided me with what I believe are important insights.

I have been on innumerable operational sites both onshore and offshore and on so many you are greeted with signs saying "Act safe", or "Think safe" or similar. These things are important, of course, but they're not sufficient on their own. Imagine if there was an injury and you told the health and safety inspector "we had lots of notices around and we had told them to be careful." You'd be in court faster than you could say "he should have been more careful." You'd be found guilty of not having provided a safe place of work.

Likewise, with mental safety, it not all about the potential injured party protecting themselves. There are wider responsibilities.

Rifleman Mitchell Matthews was found dead in July 2020 in his barracks. Suicide is suspected. His wife, Katy, was juggling being a newly qualified nurse with working on a COVID-19 ward and childcare for their five year old daughter. Mitchell sought to get some understanding from his superiors so he could be available on occasion to collect his daughter from school. He was allegedly told to "man up"[69]. A few weeks earlier a friend of his had committed suicide. Nathan's mother Alison said "The Army treats these deaths as if they are not connected. How can they not be when you have two boys, who were mates, in the same company of the same regiment taking their lives within weeks of each other? It is a massive failure of a duty of care. The Army really needs to start addressing the problem of suicide within its ranks. It is nothing short of a disgrace."

An Army spokesman said: "Rifleman Mitchell Matthews's death was a tragedy and our thoughts remain with his family and friends at this difficult time. We strive to be a modern employer, and the Army takes the health and wellbeing of its personnel very seriously and provides

---

[69] Army told my hero husband to 'man up' before he took his own life, Daily Mirror, 20th September 2020.

a wide range of support from flexible working to mental health services."

A commitment to mental safety might help.

7. Snowflakes

Another popular expression is "snowflake". By this I don't mean a flake of snow, but rather a term of abuse.

The Oxford English Dictionary defines it as:

"Originally and chiefly U.S. (usually derogatory and potentially offensive). Originally: a person, esp. a child, regarded as having a unique personality and potential. Later: a person mockingly characterized as overly sensitive or easily offended, esp. one said to consider himself or herself entitled to special treatment or consideration."

It's this later definition that is in common parlance. The concept is that people need to be less sensitive and more resilient as discussed under "Be strong". Although people should be as tough as possible and not overly-sensitive, it's important that the entire onus isn't laid on the individual at risk any more than is the case in other areas of safety. A mental injury is an injury as much as a physical injury.

It's just as inappropriate to blame the victim of a mental safety incident as it is to blame a victim of a mugger.

8. Normalisation of deviance

Neil Armstrong walked on the moon on 1969. The rockets used for the Apollo programme were single-use devices. Some three years before that, the need for a partially reusable space craft was identified by the US Air Force and NASA. The result was the space shuttle, which flew 135 missions from 1981 to 2011.

On 28th January 1986, the space shuttle *Challenger* was launched. 73 seconds into its flight it catastrophically disintegrated leading to the death of all seven crew members including a civilian school teacher.

The shuttle was fitted with two solid rocket boosters (SRBs) for take off. The SRBs were manufactured in sections with the joints closed by O-ring seals. Prior to the launch low temperatures were experienced which led to failure of an O-ring. The failure caused a breach in the SRB joint, allowing pressurised burning gas from the solid rocket motor to reach the outside and impinge on the adjacent SRB aft field joint attachment hardware and external fuel tank. This led to the separation of the right-hand SRB's aft field joint attachment and the structural failure of the external tank. Aerodynamic forces broke up the orbiter.

An investigation was established under the leadership of William P. Rogers. It found that as early as 1977 NASA managers had not only known about the flawed O-ring, but that it had the potential for catastrophe. The commission therefore concluded the disaster was "an accident rooted in history"[70]. They identified many technical and cultural issues in NASA.

Following this Diane Vaughan, an American sociologist, coined the expression "normalisation of deviance."[71] She defined it as a process where a clearly unsafe practice comes to be considered normal if it does not immediately cause a catastrophe: "a long incubation period [before a final disaster] with early warning signs that were either misinterpreted, ignored or missed completely."

This takes us to the principle of risk. Risk is a widely used expression. In safety, it's defined as:

The consequence of an event x its probability

Because there is only a possibility that a bad thing will occur if we do wrong, people will tend to say "that went OK, so I can do the same again." That, of course, is to misunderstand the concept of risk. If you do keep on doing a bad thing you will come a cropper.

Let's think about the Associate Director at Company A in our case study. He thought it was acceptable to take information from the client at face value. It's likely that this represented his core standards from his past behaviour. Furthermore, his action was endorsed by his management. Hence, a new low standard was established. Company A is an engineering consultancy. Do they apply the same standard to

---

[70] Report of the Presidential Commission on the Space Shuttle Challenger Accident, 1986.
[71] The Challenger Launch Decision: Risky Technology, Culture and Deviance at NASA, Diane Vaughan, 1996.

technical data from the client? If not, why the difference? Does it matter less that someone can be mentally damaged than if they can be physically damaged?

If you permit normalisation of deviance, you will not be demonstrating that everyone has the right to return home mentally undamaged.

9.   Cognitive dissonance

Leon Festinger was a social psychologist. In the summer of 1954 he read a story in his local newspaper headlined "Prophecy from planet Clarion[72] call to city: flee that flood."

The warning was from Dorothy Martin (1900–1992), a Chicago housewife who experimented with automatic writing. She'd previously been involved with L. Ron Hubbard's Dianetics movement, and incorporated ideas from what is now known as Scientology. Martin headed a cult whose members had given up jobs, possessions and families in the expectation they would be evacuated on a flying saucer which would rescue the group of true believers. Martin had received messages that the world would end in a great flood before dawn on 21st December 1954.

Festinger infiltrated the sect to see what would happen when the prophecy was proved untrue. He noticed that its members made little effort to persuade other people that the end was near. Salvation was reserved for them, the chosen few. On the morning of 21st December 1954, Martin received the message: "At the hour of midnight you shall be put into parked cars and taken to a place where ye[73] shall be put aboard a porch [flying saucer]."

The excited group settled in to await their rescue. At 11:15 p.m. Martin received a message telling the group to put on their coats and prepare. Midnight came and nothing happened. At 12:05 a.m. one of the group noticed another clock in the room read 11:55 p.m. They agreed it wasn't yet midnight. At 12:10 a.m. there was a message from the aliens: The flying saucers are delayed. It seems even extra-

---

[72] The planet Clarion is allegedly on the other side of our sun (or depending where you research, the moon) and so (conveniently) can't be seen from the Earth. I'm not quite sure how that works in astronomical terms.

[73] It's interesting that extra-terrestrials use medieval English. Possibly they read Chaucer and Shakespeare.

---

terrestrials have problems with traffic. At 12:15 a.m. the telephone rang several times. It was journalists calling to check if the world had ended yet. (You imagine they might know if it had). At 4:00 a.m. one of the believers said "I've burned every bridge. I've turned my back on the world. I can't afford to doubt. I have to believe." At 4:45 a.m. Martin got another message. God had decided to spare the Earth. Together, the small group of believers had spread so much "light" on this night that the Earth had been saved. At 4:50 a.m. there was one last message from above: The aliens wanted the good news "to be released immediately to the newspapers." Armed with this new mission, the believers informed all the local papers and radio stations before daybreak.

After the failed prediction, Martin was threatened with arrest and left Chicago. She later founded the Association of Sananda and Sanat Kumara under the name Sister Thedra.

"A man with a conviction is a hard man to change." So opens Leon Festinger's account of these events in his seminal work "When Prophecy Fails"[74], first published in 1956. "Tell him you disagree and he turns away, show him facts or figures and he questions your sources. Appeal to logic and he fails to see your point."

Festinger called this "Cognitive dissonance". When reality clashes with our deepest convictions, we'd rather recalibrate reality than amend our world view. Not only that, we become even more rigid in our beliefs than before. This generally – but not always – is with reference to our strongly held beliefs, such as politics or religion. We can be more accommodating when it comes to trivia. The big issues tend to define who we are and what our identity is.

An oft-quoted example of this is smoking despite knowing that tobacco can lead to cancer.

This can affect attitudes to safety and perhaps especially mental safety.

---

[74] In his book, Festinger changed the name of the "prophet" from Dorothy Martin to Marian Keech and relocated the event from Chicago to Michigan.

10. Won't you be taken advantage of?

We all know the scenario. Management introduce a benefit. Staff take it as being a right or even worse misuse it. Years ago in the UK civil service there was a working assumption that staff would be absent for a certain number of days a year due to sickness. Before long this was seen to be an additional leave allowance, only obviously not booked in advance with the employer!

Is the same sort of abuse awaiting employers if we pursue mental safety?

We know already that many stress-related absences are difficult to divide into work-related and non-work-related causes. Responsible organisations will seek to examine events to determine what the work-related aspects are and investigate them to identify the causes and the lessons arising. That won't change but it will require us to get more professional about it.

Obviously stress is a difficult thing to prove but if stress is reported and a valid cause (irrespective of whether it led to a stress outcome) is identified that is significant.

We have similar issues in the mainstream safety agenda. Muscular-skeletal injuries are difficult to prove but that doesn't stop us reporting and investigating them even though some of them might actually be bogus.

We need to ensure that we provide a work environment that people are content in.

CHAPTER EIGHT

DRAWING IT ALL TOGETHER

1. What do I think about companies A and B?

People ask me what I now think of Companies A and B.

The ideal thing would be to be able to say that I don't think of them at all, preferring to treat them with the contempt they have ladled out to me - but that isn't how these things work. I have been maligned and abused and this has damaged me in such a way that it's impossible for me not to think of what happened day again and again. This is quite literally mind numbing. I go to sleep tired and I wake up tired. Unfortunately you can't reboot your brain like you can a computer.

Neither company has come to terms with what they did or apologised, preferring to arrogantly pretend that they followed their procedures despite being caught bang to rights by the evidence.

But they are both companies that say they stand for so many things, including incident investigation and learning from experience. This is an outstanding case of them not living up to so many of their alleged values.

The irony is that if mental safety achieves the traction it deserves, Company A will probably try to sell its services as a consultant in the field!

2. Conclusions

So what do I conclude?

It's recognised that in terms of data, I am not comparing like with like. However, it is the best data available and my conclusions and recommendations are still valid. They are:

1. Suicides and stress events are showing no reduction over a period of 20 years.

2. There is insufficient information on the cause of suicides. In particular, in the UK there is no information on how many suicides are work-related.

3. Although there is an increased focus on mental health, this is showing no detectable improvement in stress and other frequencies or lost time.

4. Our case study shows how shallow corporate commitment to mental health can be.

5. Organisations care less about the mental health of non-employees than of employees. Hence the gig economy serves to make the problem worse.

6. Most, if not all, organisations fail to care about mental health to the same degree that they do physical safety or process safety.

7. There is a shortfall in interest in this from legislators, regulators and other stakeholders. The failure of a visible cause-consequence relationship in mental health contributes to the problem and acts as a shield to hide behind.

8. There has been a remarkable improvement in safety in the UK and many other countries since the 1970s. This has been caused by intense focus on risk and its management.

3. Recommendations

What do I recommend?

1. It must be universally accepted and demonstrated that all workers have a right to go home mentally undamaged in the same way they deserve to go home physically undamaged.

2. We should start to talk about mental health and safety and not just mental health.

3. Mental safety should adopt many of the principles that have a demonstrated track record of success in physical safety in addition to the aspects of mental health.

4. Legislators, regulators and other stakeholders need to demonstrate that they care about mental safety and ensure it gets focus equivalent to that applied in other forms of safety.

5. Adoption of the Shamrock Model will demonstrate that mental safety is equal to physical safety and process safety.

6. Work-related suicides need to be measured.

However, if there is one word which sums up what all organisations ought to have, it is quite simply:

Integrity

Printed in Great Britain
by Amazon

74135823R00061